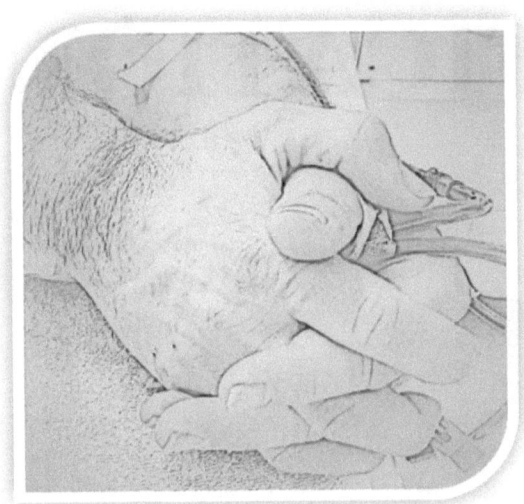

BLOOD PURIFICATION

Dialysis interventions to achieve required blood composition changes in men by its artificial machine purification on the principles of diffusion/dialysis, convection (membrane filtration), adsorption and osmosis.

Extracorporeal elimination treatment involves a variety of modes of treatment that aim to modify blood composition and properties in order to positively influence the disease process in terms of cure or at least stopping the ongoing process or stabilizing the patient's clinical condition. A substantial part of these methods of extra-body elimination treatment are methods that belong to the area of Renal Replacement Therapy (RRT). The basic physical and chemical principles underpinning the successful clinical application of these methods include diffusion and molecular diffusion, convection (membrane filtration), adsorption and osmosis (molecular water diffusion). The first part of the work (Chapter 2) deals with a detailed description of these physical and chemical principles after defining and proposing the classification of extracorporeal (extra-body) elimination treatment methods (Chapter 1). The third chapter deals with the description of basic RRT methods, namely hemodialysis, hemofiltration and hemodiafiltration with a focus on the description of the technological assumptions as well as the clinical questions of the successful application of these methods in practice. Chapter 4 focuses on issues related to Continuous Renal Replacement Therapy, its various modalities, and its use in critically ill patients with acute kidney injury and multiorgan failure. The penultimate Chapter 5 is devoted to detoxification artificial hepatic supportive therapy, hepatic or liver dialysis from a wider perspective, with an aspect of the basic distribution of these methods to the nonbiological and biological support of the liver and a short description of some of the methodologies from the group. The last chapter briefly describes methods of membrane plasma separation, immunoadsorption, and LDL apheresis, focusing on the description of areas of their potential use.

BLOOD PURIFICATION

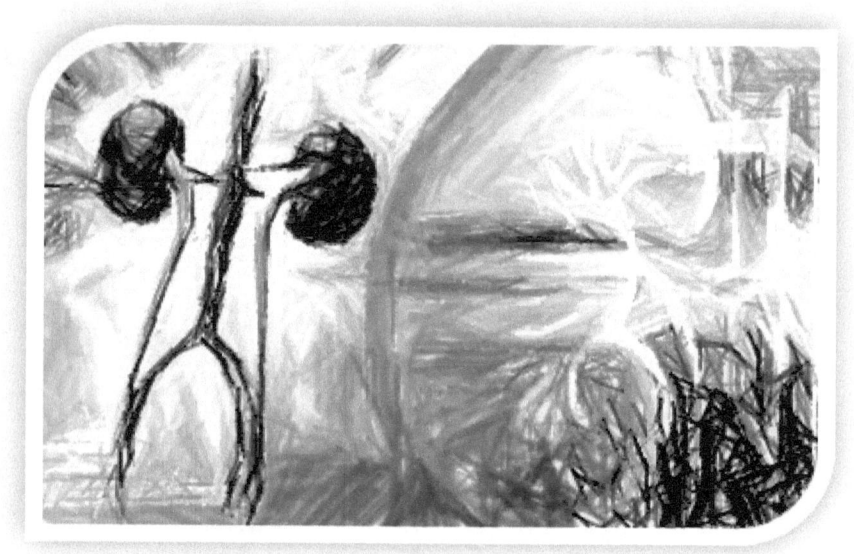

Specialized Work

By

Lubomir POLASCIN, MD

On

EXTRACORPOREAL ELIMINATION TREATMENT

Dialysis interventions to achieve required blood composition changes in men by its artificial machine purification on the principles of diffusion/dialysis, convection (membrane filtration), adsorption and osmosis.

Text Copyright © Lubomir Polascin 2019

All Rights Reserved

The First Author's Own Release. US English Edition. Bratislava, Rovinka © Lubomir Polascin, March 2019.

Author's Statement and Disclaimer.

This specialized work of Lubomir POLASCIN is subject to copyright. All rights are reserved, whether the whole or part of the book is concerned, specifically the rights of translation, reprinting, reuse, recitation, broadcasting, reproduction in any physical and non-physical way, and transmission or information storage and retrieval, electronic adaptation, or by similar or dissimilar ways now known or hereafter made usable in the future.

No one part of this book may be translated into other languages, reproduced or utilized in any form, by any means electronic or mechanical, including photocopying, recording, other copying, or by any information storage and retrieval system, without permission in writing form of the author of this work.

Any use of general descriptive names, registered names, trademarks, service marks, etc. in this book does not imply, even in the absence of a specific statement, that such names are exempt from the relevant protective laws and regulations and therefore free for general use.

I, as the author obviously assume all information in this book is believed to be true and accurate at the date of writing. The author does not give a warranty, express or implied, with respect to the information contained herein or for any mistakes or omissions that may have been made.

This work is not under any circumstances intended to be, and should not be considered, a substitute for any health or any different medical or other advice. Therapy for the conditions described in this material is highly dependent on individual patient conditions. As this work of mine is meant to offer accurate information with respect to the subject covered and to be current as of the time it was written, research and knowledge about medical and health issues are constantly evolving and dose schedules for medications are being revised continually, with new side effects recognized and accounted for on a regular basis. Readers of this book must therefore always read any medical or pharmaceutical product information and clinical procedures with the most up-to-date published product information and data sheets provided by the manufacturers of the products, summary of the product's characteristics and the most recent codes of conduct and safety regulation. The author of this book makes no representations or warranties to anybody, express or implied, as for the accuracy or completeness of this information provided. Without limiting the foregoing, the author is not liable to accept, and expressly disclaim, any responsibility for any liability, loss or risk that may be claimed or incurred because of the appropriate or inappropriate use and/or application of any of the content of this work.

The statements, opinions, and data contained in this book are those of the individual authors cited. The author has exerted every reasonable effort to ensure that drug selection and dosage set forth in this book of mine are in accord with current recommendations, guidelines, and practice at the time of writing. But having current progress in view of ongoing research, changes in various government regulations and the constant flow of information relating to any therapy and adverse reactions, the reader of this book is urged to check the package inserts for each drug for any change in indications and dosage and for added warning and precautions. This is extremely important when the recommended agent is a new one and/or infrequently used.

ABSTRACT

POLASCIN, Lubomir: Blood Purification. Extracorporeal (Extra-Body) elimination (excretion) treatment/therapy. Dialysis interventions to achieve required blood composition changes in men by its artificial machine purification on the principles of diffusion/dialysis, convection (membrane filtration), adsorption and osmosis. **[Specialized work in the field of Nephrology and Dialysis]. The First Author's Own Release. US English Edition. Bratislava, Rovinka © Lubomir Polascin, March 2019.**

Extracorporeal (extra-body) elimination (excretion) treatment/therapy involves a variety of modes of treatment that aim to modify blood composition and properties in order to positively influence the disease process in terms of cure or at least stopping the ongoing process or stabilizing the patient's clinical condition. A substantial part of these methods of extra-body elimination treatment are methods that belong to the area of Renal Replacement Therapy (RRT). The basic physical and chemical principles underpinning the successful clinical application of these methods include diffusion and molecular diffusion, convection (membrane filtration), adsorption and osmosis (molecular water diffusion). The first part of the work (Chapter 2) deals with a detailed description of these physical and chemical principles after defining and proposing the classification of extracorporeal (extra-body) elimination treatment methods (Chapter 1). The third chapter deals with the description of basic RRT methods, namely hemodialysis, hemofiltration and hemodiafiltration with a focus on the description of the technological assumptions as well as the clinical questions of the successful application of these methods in practice. Chapter 4 focuses on issues related to Continuous Renal Replacement Therapy, its various modalities, and its use in critically ill patients with acute kidney injury and multiorgan failure. The penultimate Chapter 5 is devoted to detoxification artificial hepatic supportive therapy, hepatic or liver dialysis from a wider perspective, with an aspect of the basic distribution of these methods to the nonbiological and biological support of the liver and a short description of some of the methodologies from the group. The last chapter briefly describes methods of membrane plasma separation, immunoadsorption, and LDL apheresis, focusing on the description of areas of their potential use.

Keywords: adoption, anticoagulation, artificial hepatic or liver supportive treatment, BAL, acetate-free biofiltration, biologic support of the liver, citrate, CRRT, RRT, dialysis membrane, dialysis machine, dialysis solution, dialysate, dialyzer, diffusion, molecular diffusion, hemofiltration, hemodialysis, hemodiafiltration, heparin, immunoadsorption, continuous renal replacement therapy, convection, membrane filtration, membrane plasma separation, molecular water diffusion, substituent, substitute, substitution solution, non-biologic liver support, osmosis, paired filtration dialysis, paired filtration, liver dialysis, hepatic dialysis, plasmapheresis, Prometheus, MARS, reverse osmosis, SPAD, single pass albumin dialysis.

Preface

Extracorporeal (extra-body) elimination therapy/treatment as a part of Renal Replacement Therapy (RRT) was originally designed especially for treatment to replace renal function. It is a summary of the methods, also called blood-purifying methods, aimed at changing the composition and characteristics of the blood where there has been major acute or chronic failure of kidney functioning.

In terms of time and duration, RRT may be carried out either intermittently or continuously. Intermittent methodologies have found their application primarily in chronical (long-term) ill patients as well as in some of their modifications (e.g., short-term daily dialysis) in acute ill ones. The continuous methodologies are intended primarily for hemodynamically unstable patients and thus find their place in acute renal failure and multiorgan failure. Discovering methods in this cohort of patients even more effective is at its very start. There is, e.g., Renal Bio-Replacement Therapy (RBT).

The RRT methodologies themselves cannot replace all kidney functions or replace them completely. Therefore, the long-term patients with kidney (renal) failure need in addition to direct changes in the composition and characteristics of the blood also other supportive medical therapy. It mainly consists of the treatment of concomitant renal anemia (typically normocyte and normochromic) and a correction of the concomitant mineral bone disorder, but also to some other areas, as well as for dietary treatment, fluid intake and overall management of the cardiovascular disorders with renal failure.

In addition to the replacement of renal function, efforts are also made using the technical development of methods that directly change the composition and characteristics of the blood, also replacing the functions of other organs. In the first place, this is a substitute for hepatic failure (Mars and Prometheus Systems). Some afferent methodologies could help in case of certain impaired metabolic functions (e.g., severe lipoprotein disorders) and the elimination of etiological factors of some diseases (e.g., myasthenia) and the like ones.

The area of this treatment gradually permeates the narrow boundaries of the nephrology specialization and enters other areas of medicine. It becomes progressively a separate comprehensive complex of methods aimed at directly altering the composition and characteristics of the blood.

Content

Abstract. 0..1
Preface. 0 4
List of abbreviations and symbols. 0..10
Introduction. 0 13
1   Definition and classification. 0..15
2   Basic physical and chemical principles. 0 26
2.1   Diffusion and Molecular Diffusion.. 0 26
2.2   Convection (Membrane Filtration). 0................................39
2.3   Adsorption.. 0..49
2.4   Osmosis (Molecular Water Diffusion). 0 55
2.4.1   Reverse Osmosis. 0...60
3   Hemodialysis, Hemofiltration, and Hemodiafiltration. 0........65
3.1   Basic Principles. 0 65
3.2   Factors affecting the clearance of the solutes. 0 70
3.3   Ultrafiltration during hemodialysis. 0 73
3.4   High-Efficiency and 77
3.4.1   Highly effective (high efficacy) hemodialysis (...............77
3.4.2   „High-Flux..78
3.5   Hemofiltration and Hemodiafiltration. 0 79
3.5.1   Acetate Free Biofiltration (AFB). 0................................81
3.5.2   Paired Filtration Dialysis (PFD). 0 82
3.5.3   HFR Online. 0...83
3.6   Dialysis Membranes. 0 83
3.6.1   Cellulose-based dialysis membranes. 0 84
3.6.2   Dialysis membranes with synthetic polymers. 0 86
3.6.3   Reactions to dialysis membranes. 0................................88
3.6.4   Biocompatibility of Dialysis Membranes. 0....................90
3.7   Dialyzers. 0..92
3.8   Dialysis device (machine, monitor). 0...............................96
3.9   Dialysis solutions. 0...100
4   Continuous Renal Replacement Therapy (CRRT). 0 106
4.1   Parameters used in CRRT.. 0..110
4.2   Vascular access for the implementation of CRRT.. 0 111
4.3   Membranes and ultrafiltration achieved in CRRT.. 0 112
4.4   Dialysis and replacement solutions for CRRT.. 0 114

4.5 Anticoagulation during CRRT.. 0 116
4.5.1 Heparin (unfractionated heparin). 0 117
4.5.2 Low-molecular heparins (LMWH), fractionated. 0 119
4.5.3 Implementation of CRRT without anticoagulation. 0 119
4.5.4 Regional anticoagulants with sodium citrate. 0 120
4.5.5 Other options for anticoagulation in CRRT.. 0 122
4.6 Possible complications in CRRT.. 0 123
5 Hepatic dialysis – detoxifying artificial hepatic supportive therapy. 0 125
5.1 Non-biological liver support. 0 126
MARS – Molecular adsorption recirculating system [Molecular Adsorbent Recirculating System]. 0 129
SPAD - Dialysis with a Single Pass of Albumin. 0 130
Prometheus System®.. 0 131
5.2 Biological Liver Support. 0 131
6 Other methods of extracorporeal (extra-body) elimination treatment. 0 135
List of used literature. 0 141

LIST OF ABBREVIATIONS AND SYMBOLS

AFB	Acetate Free biofiltration
ALF	Acute liver failure - Acute hepatic failure
APD	Automated Peritoneal Dialysis
AVF	Arterio-Venous Fistula (artificial shunt)
BAL	Bioartificial Liver
CAPD	Continuous (Continual) Ambulatory (Outpatient) Peritoneal Dialysis
CAVH	Continual Arterial-Venous Hemofiltration
CAVHD	Continual Arterial-Venous Hemodialysis
CCPD	Continual Cyclic Peritoneal Dialysis
CFPD	Continual Flow Peritoneal Dialysis
CKD-MBD	Chronic Kidney Disease – Mineral Bone Disease
CRRT	Continual Renal Replacement Therapy
CVVH	Continual Vena-Venous Hemofiltration

CVVHD	Continual Vena-Venous Hemodialysis
CVVHDF	Continual Vena-Venous Hemodiafiltration
ESA	Erythropoiesis Stimulating Agent
ESKD	End-Stage Kidney Disease
ESRD	End Stage Renal Disease
HD	Hemodialysis
HDF	Hemodiafiltration
HF	Hemofiltration
IPD	Intermittent Peritoneal Dialysis
KFR	Kidney Function Replacement
KTx	Kidney Transplantation = Renal Transplantation
LDL	Low-Density Lipoproteins
LMWH	Low Molecular Weight Heparin
LNFO	Abbreviation in the Slovak Language for Kidney Function Replacement
LSD	Liver Support Device
NIPD	Night Intermittent Peritoneal Dialysis

NMC	National Medical Care
NTx	Kidney transplantation = Renal Transplantation
OCPD	Optimized Cyclic Peritoneal Dialysis
OLT	Orthotopic Liver Transplantation
ONL	Abbreviation in the Slovak Language for Kidney Replacement Therapy
PFD	Paired Filtration Dialysis
PTFE	Polytetrafluoroethylene
RBT	Renal Bioartificial Therapy
RRT	Renal Replacement Therapy
S	Sieving coefficient
SPAD	Single Pass Albumin Dialysis
TMP	Transmembrane Pressure
TPD	Tidal Peritoneal Dialysis
UF	Ultrafiltration

INTRODUCTION

I have mentioned already in this specialized book of mine in the field of nephrology; I deal with the methods of extracorporeal (extra-body) elimination treatment/therapy that largely falls within the area of the *Renal Replacement Therapy*.

It is not my ambition to cover, in this specialized work, the whole issue of the Renal Replacement Therapy, which would not, to a large extent, permit the type and expected usual range of this work. Therefore, in this book of mine I do not deal with issues such as the history of RRT, aspects of the caregiver care for extra-body (extracorporeal) elimination treatment, vascular access management and its complications (AVF, PTFE artificial graft, and possibly at the same time the sleeve or tunneled dialysis catheter, called permanent dialysis central venous catheter, temporary dialysis catheter, etc.), water treatment for dialysis, acute and chronic complications of dialysis therapy, comprehensive issues of peritoneal dialysis and kidney transplantation. Nor do I deal with issues related to long-term dialysis therapy. This includes, for example, the issue of mineral bone disease in chronic kidney/renal disease, the issue of viral hepatitis B and C types, questions regarding renal anemia and treatment with individual substances that stimulate erythropoiesis (ESA), the adequacy of dialysis treatment and the use of different anticoagulation regimes in extra-body (extracorporeal) circulation, issues of nutrition disorders by chronic kidney disease (CKD-MBD), intercultural counselling, rehabilitation and the like ones. In the work I focus on methods that directly change the composition and characteristics of the blood and related issues, with the issue of peritoneal dialysis, which can also be considered as a method of direct changing of the composition and characteristics of the blood, left aside, that it is an Intra-Body (Intracorporeal) method.

1 DEFINITION AND CLASSIFICATION

Normally, under normal circumstances, the kidneys fulfill the following basic functions:

- Eliminate (excrete) excessive amounts of sodium (Na^+), water (H_2O) and hydrogen ions H^+ (keeping the pH in the physiological range 7.40 ± 0.04);

- Remove or control the balance of other electrolytes, such as potassium (K^+), calcium (Ca^{2+}), magnesium (Mg^{2+}) and phosphates (PO_4^{2-});

- Remove waste products of metabolism - catabolites (routinely in the laboratory we test serum urea and creatinine levels, but the waste products of metabolism are of large quantities and sorts);

- Form erythropoietin in the peritubular cells of the proximal tube (tubule) of the nephron – the hormone needed to produce red blood cells in the bone marrow;

> With the help of the 1-α-hydroxylase convert 25-hydroxycholecalciferol to 1,25-dihydroxycholecalciferol and thus activate natural vitamin D to be able to act in the human body.

Extracorporeal (extra-body) elimination (excrete, excretion) therapy/treatment can replace only the first three of these functions, but it should also be noted that, even at best, they are only partially effective and are always only a partial replacement of the renal function. The replacement of the last two of the above-mentioned renal functions can largely be substituted by pharmacological means.

Renal Replacement Therapy and Extracorporeal Elimination Therapy are two intermingle sets.

Kidney transplantation as one of the options for renal replacement therapy completely supersedes all renal function and should be considered as an optimal treatment of choice for the final stage of renal disease (ESRD, ESKD). Transplanted patients experience a longer and better quality of life. However, not everyone can undergo transplantation, as patients with ESRD often suffer from significant co-morbidity, particularly vascular diseases due to mineral bone disease in chronic kidney disease (CKD-MBD). (STEDDON, 2006 p. 202)

Term Renal Replacement Therapy (RRT) or treatment can be used as a summary label for all therapeutic modalities and therapeutic procedures designed to replace renal function in cases where the kidneys of man themselves are so affected by the disease process that they are no longer capable of ensuring these renal functions in the long-term horizon.

Speaking of the basic, elimination function of kidneys with the effect on maintaining the stability of the internal body biochemical environment (homeostasis and homeokinesis), these methods of RRT could be divided in principle into three basic categories:

1. **Extracorporeal (extra-body) elimination methods**

2. **Intrabody (intracorporal) elimination methods**

3. **Kidney transplantation from an alive or dead donor (giver)**

In addition to these three categories of kidney replacement treatment, therapeutic procedures are also applied, which aim is to replace other renal function and to supplement the elimination. Some of these procedures can be defined and classified as a separate treatment method or procedure. I deal with these therapeutic procedures in the framework designation of renal function as set out in the introduction of this chapter. The following may be mentioned:

a) Treatment of secondary non-parenchymatous standard normochromic normocytic anemia by erythropoiesis-stimulating agents (ESA) associated with the treatment of possible iron deficiency by intravenous or oral iron preparations and higher doses of ascorbic acid (vitamin C) in the functional iron deficit

b) Treatment of disorders of phosphate-calcium metabolism, osteopathy, adynamic bone disease is collectively referred to as treatment of mineral bone disease in chronic kidney disease (CKD-MBD) (phosphate binders with emphasis on non-calcium contenting binders, place of preparations of calcium, natural vitamin D, active form of vitamin D – 1,25-dihydroxycholecalciferol, synthetic analogues of active vitamin D (e.g. paricalcitol), calcimimetics – medicines that increase the sensitivity for calcium concentration receptors on the surface of the main cells of the parathyroid gland to the extracellular calcium and the like).

c) Treatment of metabolic acidosis if it is not enough corrected during the treatment with elimination methods

d) Immunosuppressive treatment after kidney transplantation and overall patient management after renal transplantation

Understandably, in the implementation of the individual methods of kidney replacement treatment, we do not take any other treatment procedures designed to address, for example, acute or chronic complications of elimination therapy, secondary renal hypertension and the like, and which is not so simply unequivocally be classified in a separate block of therapeutic methods.

The following forms of elimination therapy according to Schück may be considered as a basic simple distribution of the various methods of elimination:

Blood Cleansing Methods (Blood Purification)

I. Hemoperfusion

II. Plasmapheresis

III. Replacement of renal function (RRT = Renal Replacement Therapy)

   1. Dialysis

    a. Hemodialysis

    b. Peritoneal Dialysis

2. Hemofiltration

3. Hemodiafiltration

4. Continuous methods (CAVH, CVVH, CVVHD, CVVHDF)

If I would like to look from a different perspective to the basic three types of renal replacement therapy, as I have stated in the introduction of this chapter, I could come to the next more detailed classification proposing by me myself.

I. EXTRA-BODY (EXTRACORPOREAL) ELIMINATION (EXCRETING, EXCRETION) TREATMENT / THERAPY

    a) Division by basic physical and chemical principles of the treatment:

        A. Methods using predominantly only blood-purifying options those in principle replace only some renal functions:

            1. Hemodialysis

            2. "High-Flux" and High Performance ("High-Efficiency") Hemodialysis

3. Isolated ("dry") ultrafiltration

4. Hemofiltration

    a. Predilution

    b. Postdilution

    c. High-Volume

5. Hemodiafiltration

    a. Predilution

    b. Mid-dilution

    c. Postdilution

    d. High-Volume

B. Methods using the extended 'blood-purifying' options and where appropriate, replacing other functions of another detoxification of the organism:

1. Hemoperfusion

2. Membrane Separation of Plasma (Membrane Plasma Separation) - Plasmapheresis

3. Cascade Filtration

4. Immunoadsorption and apheresis

5. Extracorporeal (Extra-Body) Supportive Treatment / Therapy of Liver (Hepatic Dialysis, Liver Dialysis)

   a. Non-Biological Liver Support

      i. Prometheus System – with the system separating fractionated plasma

      ii. MARS System – Molecular Absorption Recirculating System

      iii. SPAD – Single Pass Albumin Dialysis

   b. Biological Liver Support (bioartificial equipment)

b) Division by Time Duration:

   A. Intermittent (non-continuous, interruptive) methods

   B. Continuous (ongoing, nonstop) methods

c) Division by the Vascular Access:

A. Arterial-Venous methods

   1. Central artery catheterization (the most common femoral artery) and catheterization of the central vein

   2. Central artery catheterization (the most common femoral artery) and blood return to the peripheral vein

B. Veno-Venous methods

   1. Central venous catheter

   2. Permanent tunneled central venous catheter

   3. Implantable port

   4. Artificial Arterio-Venous Shunt with subsequent arterialization of the venous system behind the shunt (AV fistula)

   5. Arterio-Venous graft

   6. Vascular prosthesis

   7. Autologous graft

   8. Artificial graft

d) *Division according to the dialysis, eventually used replacement solution:*

    A. Bicarbonate method using bicarbonate solution (35 mmol/L of bicarbonate and 3-5 mmol/L of acetate)

    B. Lactate method using lactate solution

    C. Acetate method using acetates solution (38 mmol/L of acetate)

    D. Citrate method using a citric acid solution

II. **INTRA-BODY (INTRACORPORAL) ELIMINATION (EXCRETING, EXCRETION) TREATMENT / THERAPY**

    A. Intermittent Peritoneal Dialysis (IPD)

    B. Continuous Ambulatory / Outpatient Peritoneal Dialysis (CAPD)

    C. Automated Peritoneal Dialysis (APD)

        1. Night Intermittent Peritoneal Dialysis (NIPD)

        2. Continuous Cyclic Peritoneal Dialysis (CCPD)

3. Optimized Continuous Peritoneal Dialysis (OCPD) or PD Plus

4. Tidal ("Tidal") Peritoneal Dialysis (TPD)

D. Continuous Flow Peritoneal Dialysis (CFPD)

III. RENAL TRANSPLANTATION - KIDNEY TRANSPLANTATION (KTx, NTx) AS THE THIRD PILLAR OF THE RENAL REPLACEMENT THERAPY

A. KTx from the alive donor (giver), relatives or so-called emotional relatives

B. KTx from the dead (cadaverous) donor (giver)

2 BASIC PHYSICAL AND CHEMICAL PRINCIPLES

Essential successful use of the extracorporeal (extra-body), elimination treatment technology, is based on the knowledge and successful use of several basic physical-chemical principles that can be described as the technological principles of extracorporeal (extra-body) elimination. These are the following principles:

1. **Diffusion, Molecular Diffusion.**
2. **Convection (Membrane Filtration).**
3. **Adsorption.**
4. **Osmosis (Molecular Diffusion of Water).**

2.1 Diffusion and Molecular Diffusion

Molecular diffusion, often commonly simplified as diffusion, is a network transfer of molecules from an area with a higher concentration into an area with a lower concentration through accidental molecular movement. Despite this, Molecular Diffusion continues to occur even after this concentration's equalization. This movement demonstrates the phenomenon known as Brown's movement. This is a continuous unordered chaotic movement of particles. The phenomenon was named after Scottish botanist Robert Brown who in 1827 watched the behavior of the pollen grains in the water. This was considered proof that the pollen is alive. The true essence of this phenomenon was clarified in 1905 by Albert Einstein. It was based on the kinetic theory of substances. The molecules in the solution are constantly precipitated under the influence of heat movement, and the direction and strength of these movements are accidental, and this makes the particle position accidental. The Brown's movement can be described by statistical, mathematical methods, and the phenomenon is referred to as particle theory, it ranks among the stochastic (random) processes. (Wikipedia. The Free Encyclopedia. Molecular diffusion, 2009)

The diffusion is, therefore, a spontaneous **passive** transport of the substance from the higher concentration environment to the lower-concentration environment. Diffusion through a semi-permeable membrane is called **dialysis**. In the course of hemodialysis, catabolites from the blood through the membrane to the dialysis solution are removed from the body. Subsequently, the reverse diffusion indicates the transition of substances in the opposite direction, i.e., from the dialysis solution to the blood. For example, it applies to the correction of the acid-basic equilibrium (the transfer of the alkaline molecule from the dialysis solution to the blood). (SULKOVÁ, 2000 s. 59-60)

The semipermeable membrane allows the passage of substances of a certain molecular weight only. Substances the molecular weight of which does not prevent the passage through a semipermeable membrane shall be moved according to the concentration gradient in the case of diffusion. (TESAŘ, 2006 s. 514)

Diffusion is one of the transport phenomena or mechanisms. In principle, two types of diffusion are distinguished:

1. *Trace diffusion.*

    This is the spontaneous transfer of molecules that occur if the concentration gradient is not present in the environment. This type of diffusion can be monitored by means of marked radioactive isotopes of elements. This diffusion takes place in the conditions of equilibria (equilibrium).

2. *Chemical diffusion.*

    This diffusion occurs in the presence of concentration gradient (chemical potential) and causes the network transport of the substance. This process is described by the diffusion equation and is always an uneven process that increases the entropy of the system and leads to equilibrium. This is a spontaneous and irreversible process.

In physics and chemistry, many other types of diffusion are distinguished, such as atomic diffusion, higher described Brown's movement, collective diffusion, swirl diffusion, effusion, electron diffusion (resulting in the electricity generation), the facilitated diffusion, gas diffusion (used for isotopic separation), thermal balance, the diffusion in mathematics, Knudsen's diffusion, torque diffusion, photon diffusion, reverse diffusion, rotary diffusion, surface diffusion and more. The antibody elimination treatment molecular diffusion phenomenon, known as chemical diffusion, which is controlled by the Fick's Law was derived by Adolf Fick in 1855. (Wikipedia. The Free Encyclopedia. Molecular diffusion, 2009)

The First Fick's Law refers to the flow of diffusion in the direction of the concentration gradient by the postulation of the fact that the flow takes place from areas of high concentration to lower concentrations and its size proportionally corresponds to the concentration gradient (spatial derivative). For one-dimension equation applies

$$J = -D \frac{\partial \phi}{\partial \chi},$$

Where

- ⇒ **J** Is Diffuse flow in units [(quantity of substance) length^{-2} Time^{-1}], e.g. ($\frac{mol}{m^{-2}.s}$). **J** Indicates the quantity of a substance flowing over a small area short time interval;

- ⇒ **D** is the diffusion coefficient or diffusivity in units [length^{2} Time^{-1}], for example ($\frac{m^2}{s}$);

- ⇒ ϕ (For ideal mixtures) is the concentration in units [(amount of substance length^{-3}], for example ($\frac{mol}{m^3}$);

- ⇒ χ Is the position, the location [length], for example (m).

D proportionally corresponds to the speed of the particulate matter to the other, which depends on the temperature, the viscosity of the liquid and the particle size. The Stokes-Einstein-Sutherland equation.

$$D = \frac{k_B T}{6 \pi \eta r},$$

Where

- $\Rightarrow$ **k$_B$** Is Boltzmann's constant (1.380650424 x 10^{-23} J.k^{-1}) That we obtain by dividing Universal Gas Constant R (8.31447215 J. K^{-1}. Mol^{-1}) by the Avogadro Number A (6.0221417930 x 10^{23} Mol^{-1}); It has the same units as entropy and is named after the Austrian physics of Ludwig Boltzmann;

- $\Rightarrow$ **T** is the absolute temperature in Kelvin;

- $\Rightarrow$ π Is a mathematical constant whose value is the ratio of the circumference of the circle to its diameter (which is the ratio of the circle area to the area of the square with its diameter), and first used by William Jones in 1707 and popularized by Leonhard Euler in 1737 and is referred to as Ludolph's Number, circular constant, Archimedes constant (not Archimedes Number); it is an irrational number; thus its value cannot be accurately expressed in real numbers. It approximately equals to 3.14159265358979323846... (usually used 3.14 or 3.14159);

⇒ η Is Dynamic Media Viscosity (Fluid Resistance, "density" of the liquid) in Pascal-seconds [Pa. s], which equals [kg. m^{-1}. s^{-1}];

⇒ **r** Is Radius of the spherical particles in meters.

It can be used for the estimation of the diffuse coefficient of the globulin protein in a solution, for example, for a protein with molecular weight of 100 Kilo Dalton we get D = 10^{-10} m^2. s^{-1}, provided the "standard" density of protein is 1,2 x 10^3 Kg. m^{-3}. In aqueous solutions, diffuse coefficients for most ions are similar and at room temperature are between 0.6 x 10^{-9} To 2 x 10^{-9} m^2. s^{-1}. For biological molecules, diffuse coefficients normally are in the range of 10^{-11} up to 10^{-10} m^2. s^{-1}. (Wikipedia. The Free Encyclopedia. Fick's law of diffusion, 2009)

In two and multi-dimensional systems, we must use the operator ∇, referred to as the operator del (vector differential operator denoted by the symbol) or also called gradient operator (See in more detail Http://en.wikipedia.org/wiki/Del) which of the first derivative, bringing we obtain an equation

$$J = -D\nabla\phi$$

Driving for single-dimensional diffusion, the value of $-\frac{\partial \phi}{\partial x}$ that represents the ideal mixtures of the concentration gradient. In different chemical systems, other than ideal solutions or mixtures, is the driving force of diffusion for each of the types of the gradient of the chemical potential for the species. In this case, the first Fick's Law (for one dimension) can be entered as follows

$$J_i = -\frac{D.c_i}{R.T}\frac{\partial \mu_i}{\partial \chi},$$

Where

⇒ **i** is the index indicating the species;

⇒ **c** is the concentration [mol/M^3];

⇒ **R** is a universal gas constant [J/ (K. Mol)] (see above);

⇒ **T** is the absolute temperature [K];

⇒ **μ** is a chemical potential [J/mol].

Second Fick's Law tells us about the prediction of how the diffusion changes concentration in a given area over time:

$$\frac{\partial \phi}{\partial t} = D \frac{\partial^2 \phi}{\partial \chi^2},$$

Where

⇒ ϕ Is the concentration in units [(quantity of substance) length^{-3}], [Mol. m^{-3}];

⇒ **t** is the time [s];

⇒ **D** is the diffusion coefficient in units [length^2. Time^{-1}], [M^2. s^{-1}];

⇒ χ position, location [length], [m].

This law can be derived mathematically from the first Fick's Law. By analogy, two or more dimensions for the second Fick's Law apply the equation

$$\frac{\partial \phi}{\partial t} = D \nabla^2 \phi$$

If the diffusion coefficient is not constant, but depends on the coordinates and/or concentration, the equation is changed as

$$\frac{\partial \phi}{\partial t} = \nabla \cdot (D \nabla \phi)$$

(URSELL, 2007)

Physiologist Adolf Fick announced for the first time his currently well-known laws in 1855 as the laws governing the transport of the substance through diffusion. Fick's work was probably inspired by the earlier experiments of Thomas Graham, which, however, failed to formulate fundamental laws, making Fick become famous. Fick is likely to be motivated by the related discoveries of the Ohm law and Fourier law. (Wikipedia. The Free Encyclopedia. Fick's law of diffusion, 2009)

The Fick's experiments were dealt with the measuring of the concentrations and flows of salt flowing between two trays through water-filled tubes. It is noteworthy that Fick's work was primarily focused on the fluid diffusion because at that time the diffusion of solids was not considered generally possible. (PHILIBERT, 2005)

In biological sciences, the equation derived from the Fick's laws is often used

$$Flow = -P \cdot A \cdot ((c)_2 - (c)_1),$$

Where

- ⇒ **P** is permeability, experimentally determined "conductance" of the membrane for the substance and the temperature;

- ⇒ **A** is the surface area through which the diffusion takes place;

- ⇒ **c_2 - c_1** Concentration of a given substance along the membrane in the direction of flow (from C_1 to C_2). (Wikipedia. The Free Encyclopedia. Fick's law of diffusion, 2009)

The rate of diffusion in the case of hemodialysis depends on the coefficient of diffusion, the area of the membrane and its thickness, which the substance must pass, and the difference in blood concentrations and in the dialysis solution (i.e., concentration gradient). The temperature is also affected. Increasing the rate also the rate of diffusion increases. (SULKOVÁ, 2000 s. 60)

This dependency can be expressed by the equation

$$J_d = D_s \cdot A \cdot \frac{C_s}{d},$$

Where

⇒ D_s is the diffusion coefficient;

⇒ A is the area of the membrane;

⇒ C_s is the concentration difference;

⇒ d is the distance that the substance must pass. (SULKOVÁ, 2000 s. 60)

Its own driving force is the concentration gradient. Diffusion coefficient depends on the properties of the membrane and the characteristics of the substance, i.e., its molecular weight and the charge. The membrane makes the diffuser conditional on its understanding (pore size, their shape, and number), thickness, the degree of hydrophilia and its electrical charge. (SULKOVÁ, 2000 s. 60-61)

Substances with a small molecular weight are diffused to remove better than substances with a large molecule. The permeability of the membrane may alter the effects of proteins that are adsorbed on the membrane during the procedure, given that this changes the pore characteristics. (SULKOVÁ, 2000 s. 61)

The inverse of the diffusion coefficient is the so-called resistance to diffusion. It is the sum of three items (resistance of the stagnant layer of blood, membrane and the stagnant layer of dialysis solution). Resistance to the transport of small substances is mainly a slow-moving layer of blood along the membrane (referred to as a stagnant surface layer, "boundary layer"). This depends on the blood flow and geometric arrangement of the membrane in the dialyzer. Resistance for large molecules is mainly given by the physical and chemical properties of the membrane. The flow ratios of blood and dialysis solution are of minor importance. During dialysis the blood and dialysis solution are in constant motion, thus still maintaining the concentration and the components of diffuse resistance is reduced. (SULKOVÁ, 2000 s. 61)

Diffusion of a certain substance may be characterized by the diffusion coefficient Ko or Co (in the above equation it corresponds to the diffusion coefficient D_s). The total size of diffusion that can be achieved by certain dialyzer is referred to as CoA ("Mass transfer area coefficient," i.e., the coefficient of transmission of the substance). It specifies the maximum actual achievable clearance value for the substance. (SULKOVÁ, 2000 s. 61)

2.2 Convection (Membrane Filtration)

The concept of convection generally indicates the movement of molecules in liquid environments, and it represents the main way for the transfer of substances. When using the methods of the extracorporeal (extra-body) elimination treatment, it involves the transfer of substances by currents, specific process for the realignment of dissolved substances together with solvent through a semipermeable membrane (a semi-permeable diaphragm) – membrane filtration. The solutions are permeating through a membrane that is called filtration. It is, therefore, a simultaneous transport of the solvent and the solution, in our case of water and dissolved substance through the membrane. Its **driving force** is in our case **Effective Pressure Gradient** on the membrane.

Filtration is a mechanical or physical activity that uses the medium through which the fluid passes (e.g., membrane) but fixed, or the dissolved components of the solution do not pass through this medium. It should also be stressed that separation is not complete and depends on the size and shape of the pores, the thickness of the medium (or membrane) as well as the mechanisms that occur during filtration.

Phenomenon used in methods of the extracorporeal (extra-body) elimination treatment can be described as the **Sieving**, as the filter medium uses a single-layer membrane. In a narrower sense, as a filtration, a plot is used to use a multi-layer medium.

The Ultrafiltration (**UF**) is denoted by membrane filtration, which uses the hydrostatic pressure to the semipermeable membrane. The dissolved substances are depending on their molecular weight of the membrane, while water and some substances pass through the membrane. Ultrafiltration is not fundamentally different from microfiltration or nanofiltration as to the question of the size of the molecules retained. In microfiltration, the size of the microfilter membrane pores from 0.1 to 10 micrometers (μm) is typical. Nanofiltration is used in solutions with a very small proportion of dissolved substances, such as drinking water and surface water. Purpose is the softening (removal of polyvalent cations) and removal of disinfectants, both natural and synthetic organic substances. It is also used for partial demineralization (removal of the mineral ions) and the desalination of water.

Different modes of ultrafiltration include:

1. *Pressurized system or configuration with a pressurized container.*

   The transmembrane pressure (TMP) is applied when the permeation remains at atmospheric pressure. Pressure vessels are generally standardized and allow a membrane system to function independently.

2. *Submersible system.*

   The membranes are immersed in containers with the solution for filtering at the atmospheric pressure. The pressure on entering the containers is limited to Pressure Column (filter solution). The other option is that the TMP is created by the pressure created by negative pressure on the side of the permeate.

Ultrafiltration, as well as other methods of filtration, can be used continuously or in batches.

The membranes in filtration can have different geometry:

1. *Spiral wined module*

   It consists of large, attached layers of membrane and support material rolled around the tube that maximizes surface area. It is not so expensive but is more sensitive to pollution.

2. *Tubular membrane*

The solution for filtration passes through the nucleus of the membrane, and the permeation is collected on the outside of the membrane, between the membrane and the cover. It is generally used for liquids of very viscous or poor quality.

3. *Hollow filament membrane ("Hollow Fiber Membrane")*

The modules contain several small (diameter 0.6 to 2 mm) tubes or fibers. The filtration solution is carried out through open fiber cores, and the permeation is collected in the supply area around the fibers. Filtration can be carried out either "from inside out" or "outside the bottom."

In biology, ultrafiltration is conducted through the blood and filtrate in the Renal or Bowman Sac (Case) in the kidneys. Bowman sac contains a dense network of capillaries called Glomerulus. Blood flows through these capillaries through a wide afferent arteriole and leaves them through a narrower efferent arteriole. The blood pressure inside these capillaries is high because

> ➢ The renal artery contains blood under high pressure with which it enters the Glomeruli through a short afferent arteriole;

> ➢ The Efferent Arteriole has a lower diameter than the afferent arteriole.

This pressure represses small molecules such as water, glucose, amino acids, chloride sodium, and urea through a filter, from blood in glomerular arterioles through the basal membrane of Bowman sac into the inside of the **Nephron**. This type of high-pressure filter filtration is called ultrafiltration. The fluid thus created is called glomerular filtrate.

The glomerular pressure is approximately 75 millimeters of mercury (mmHg) (it equals to 10 kPa). It acts as osmotic pressure (approx. 30 mmHg, 4.0 kPa) and hydrostatic pressure (20 mmHg, 2.7 kPa) of the solutes found in the housing compartment. The difference in pressures is called **effective pressure** (25 mmHg, 3.3 kPa).

As well as diffusion, filtration can take place in both directions – from the blood to the dialysis solution, but also reversed from the dialysis solution to the blood. This is then the so-called Reverse Filtration („Back Filtration ").

Hemofiltration indicates a medical technology that eliminates excessive amounts of solutes and water from the body safely, predictably and effectively. Patients suffer from transmission. It eliminates excessive amounts of solutes and water and helps maintain fluid balance in the patient or euvolemia.

After an hour, this method can remove approximately 500 mL of excess fluid, but the average is 250 mL per hour. The liquid being removed is isotonic, and therefore it eliminates approximately 3.2 g of sodium per liter of liquid removed. (CONSTANZO, 2007)

The quantity of substance removed by convection during filtration determines the product quantity of the filtrate and concentration of the substance in the filtrate. This concentration determines the product concentration of the substance in the blood (C_B) and the value of the sieving coefficient (S). (SULKOVÁ, 2000 s. 61)

Factors that influence the speed of the filtrate include the

> ➢ Hydraulic permeability of the membrane (K_f),

- Membrane area (**A**),
- Effective Pressure Gradient on the membrane (**Δp-δπ**),

What can be expressed by the equation:

$$J_c = Q_F \cdot C_B \cdot S = K_f \cdot A \cdot (\Delta P - \Delta \pi) \cdot C_B \cdot S$$

(SULKOVÁ, 2000 s. 61),

Where

⇒ J_c Is the speed of transport of the removed substance;

⇒ Q_F Is the speed of the filtrate flow;

⇒ C_B Is the concentration of the substance in the blood;

⇒ **S** is the sieving coefficient;

⇒ K_f is the hydraulic permeability of the membrane;

⇒ **A** Is the area of the membrane;

⇒ **(Δp −δπ)** represents the Effective Pressure Gradient on the membrane (difference in the sum of the pressure changes on one side of the membrane and the sum of pressure changes on the other side of the membrane).

Hydraulic permeability of the membrane (**K_f**) is the amount of ultrafiltrate per unit of time for a single hydrostatic pressure operating on a membrane with the unit area. The ultrafiltration characteristics of the dialyzer usually *Ultrafiltrate Coefficient* (**U_f**), the value of which is given in [mL/mmHg/h]. It is, therefore, the hydraulic permeability transferred to the specific area of the dialyzer (hydraulic permeability multiplied by the surface membrane). Size of ultrafiltrate is the main criterion for the ("Low-Flux") and high permeable dialyzer ("High-Flux "), although this division is not completely expressible because it does not look at the size of the sieving coefficient. The high ultrafiltration coefficient can also be achieved in the membrane with small pores, if the area of the membrane of the dialyzer is sufficiently large or very thin, or it will have many pores. However, in practice, the normal designation of high-permeable dialysis means dialysis with high ultrafiltration and the sieving coefficient. (SULKOVÁ, 2000 s. 62)

Sieving coefficient (***S***) is defined as the concentration ratio of the substance (i.e., "membrane") and concentrations of the same substance in plasma (i.e., before the membrane "). For small molecules equals one. From a certain relative molecular weight, it starts to fall. Low-permeable membranes have a permeability of substances with a relative molecular weight of 1.000 to 10.000 significantly limited and larger molecules do not release at all. High permeable membranes have a sieving coefficient for molecules with a size of 1.000 close to one and are also released Relative Molecular weight of 10.000. The hydraulic permeability and the sieving coefficient for the substance removed are specific for each membrane because they are dependent on the size of the pores and their number of units of the area. (SULKOVÁ, 2000 s. 62)

Pressure-acting on the membrane is referred to as an *Efficient Pressure Gradient on Membrane* (**Δp-δπ**), and it is the driving force of convection or ultrafiltration. For water solution, it is true that at zero pressure gradient, ultrafiltration is zero and linear rises along with increasing effective pressure on the membrane. However, the protein solution is characterized by two differences:

1. ***Move to the right.***

    The ultrafiltration does not occur until the hydrostatic pressure gradient does not exceed the oncotic pressure and the relationship is linear only after certain pressure values.

2. *Concentration Polarization.*

When further pressure increases, the ultrafiltration is no longer increased, and further increases by pressure gradient are no longer affected. This is because by the effects of pressure forces proteins are driven to the membrane that they cannot pass through, thereby complaining about their own convection transport. The size of the maximum possible ultrafiltration is the function of protein concentration and blood flow. (SULKOVÁ, 2000 s. 62)

For individual types of extracorporeal (extra-body) elimination treatment methods the relative task of diffusion and convection differs. Hemodialysis mainly uses the proportion of convection to the catabolites are relatively small, and their relative importance depends on the size of the molecule. Substances with a small molecule are removed by diffusion, and the convection contributes to their overall elimination in a limited measure. The convection and its importance for the total quantity removed are increasing with the larger molecules. The exception is small molecules if they are contained in the blood and in dialysis solution at higher concentrations (sodium). The concentration gradient is small, and the removal takes place mainly by convection. (SULKOVÁ, 2000 s. 63)

2.3 Adsorption

For membranes with hydrophobic properties, the physical-chemical principle accesses the transfer of substances through the dialysis membrane in some proteins and the adsorption phenomenon. In some methods of extracorporeal (extra-body) elimination treatment the adsorption to the membrane is significantly involved in the total removed quantity of the substance during the procedure. For example, the following substances are removed by adsorption:

- Albumin
- Bilirubin
- Amino Acids
- Myoglobin
- Fibrin
- Fragments of the activated complement system
- Some cytokines
- β_2-Microglobulin. (SULKOVÁ, 2000 s. 64)

Adsorption is a process that occurs when the gas or liquid solution accuses on the surface of a solid substance or liquid (adsorbent) where it forms a film of molecules or atoms (adsorbate). This is a process that differs from absorption, where the substance changes into a liquid or solid substance from the solution. The term sorption includes both processes until the term desorption is a reverse process.

Adsorption occurs in many natural physical, biological and chemical systems and is widely used in industrial applications such as activated charcoal, synthetic cuttings, and water purification.

Like surface tension, adsorption is the result of surface energy. In the fixed material, all binding requirements (ionic, convenctical, metallic) atoms, of which the material consists, filled with other material atoms. However, the atoms on the surface of the adsorbent are not completely covered by other adsorbent atoms and can, therefore, attract adsorbates. Exact nature of the partial binding depends on the detailed properties of the parent material, but the adsorption process is commonly referred to as *Physisorption* (characterized by weak van der Waals's forces) or *Chemisorption* (characterized by covalent ties).

Adsorption is usually described using isothermal curves. *Isotherm* is the amount of adsorbate per adsorbent as a function of its pressure (in the case of gas) or concentration (in the case of fluid) at a constant temperature. The adsorbed quantity is almost always normalized by the material adsorbent for the purpose of allowing comparisons of different materials.

According to the nature of the forces involved in the adsorbent and adsorbate, we distinguish three types of adsorption: *Physical* (molecular, non-polar), *Electrical* (Ionic and chemical) and *Chemisorption*. For physical adsorption with the adsorbates linked to the surface by the weak Van der Waal forces, with the polar adsorption by electrostatic coulomb's arterial forces and for the chemisorption adsorbates are bound by very strong forces of similar chemical custody.

Adsorbents are usually used in the form of spherical pellets, rods, strips or monoliths with hydrodynamic diameters between 0.5 and 10 mm. They must have high abrasive resistance, high thermal stability, and small pore diameters, achieving high exposure surface and thus the high surface capacity of the adsorption. Adsorbents must also have a fine porous structure that allows faster transport. Most adsorbents can be divided into three classes.

1. Oxygen-containing compounds are typically hydrophilic and polar, and these are materials of silicone gel and zeolites.

2. Carbon-containing compounds are typically hydrophobic and non-polar, and these are materials such as activated charcoal and graphite.

3. Polymer-based compounds are polar or non-polar functional groups in the porous polymer matrix.

Silicone gel is chemically inert, non-toxic, polar and dimensionally stable (< 400°C) amorphic form of SiO_2. It is prepared by the reaction between silicate sodium and Sulphur acid, followed by a series of subsequent processing processes. After these treatment methods have been done different pore sizes and different distribution are present. It is used to desiccation air or other gases and adsorption of heavy (polar) hydrocarbons from the air.

Zeolites are natural or synthetic crystalline aluminosilicates, which have a repeating porous mesh and release water at a high temperature. Zeolites are from their Nature of the polar. They are produced by hydrothermal synthesis of fluosilicate sodium or another silicate in an autoclave with a subsequent exchange of ions with certain cations such as $Na^+, K^+, Ca^{2+}, NH_4^+$. Channel diameter of the zeolite cage usually ranges from 2 to 9 Å (200 to 900 pm). The ion exchange process is followed by the drying of crystals, which can be faced with a binder into the form of macroporous pellets. Zeolites with use of air drying, CO_2, CO, air separation, catalytic cracking, and catalytic synthesis and reforming a non-polar (silicate) zeolites are synthesized from aluminum-free silicates or by the dealumination of aluminum-containing oils. This process is done by saving zeolites under high steam pressures and elevated temperatures usually higher than 500°C (1000°F). These conditions interfere with the links between oxygen and aluminum, and the aluminum atoms are off from the zeolite network.

Activated charcoal is a highly porous, amorphous rigid substance consisting of microcrystals with graphite grille, which is usually prepared in the form of small pellets or powder. It is nonpolar and cheap. One of its biggest disadvantages is that it is flammable. Activated charcoal can be produced from carbon material such as coal (bituminous, sub-bituminous and lignite), peat, wood, nut packaging (e.g., coconut nut). The production process consists of two phases – carbonization and activation. The carbonization process includes drying and then heating for the purpose of separating the by-products, including other carbonates from raw materials, as well as the keeping of all the gases generated. The carbonization process is terminated by heating the material to 400 – 600 °C in an atmosphere without oxygen, which does not support incineration. The carbonized particles are "activated" by exposing the oxidation agent, usually by steaming or carbon dioxide at high temperature. This reagent burns off pores blocked by structures created during the carbonization phase, thus creating a porous, three-dimensional structure of the graphite grid. The size of pores created during activation is a function of the time that the material spends at this stage. Longer exposure times create larger pore sizes. The most popular water-phase carbonates are those based on Bitumen coal, due to their hardness, abrasion resistance, pore size distribution, and low price, but their effectiveness should be tested in each application for the purpose of determining the optimal product. Activated charcoal is used for the adsorption of organic substances and non-polar adsorbates and is usually used for wastewater treatment and waste gases. It is the broadest used adsorbent. Its usefulness comes mainly from its large micropore and mesopores and the resulting large surface area. (Wikipedia. The Free Encyclopedia. Adsorption, 2009)

The use of adsorption in the extracorporeal (extra-body) elimination treatment is also in recent times developed by the so-called HFR Online (Hemodiafiltration with ONLINE Endogenous reinfusion). The blood flows through the device, the first part of which is a filter, the filtrate generated is then transferred to the capsule with the adsorbate, and then this filtrate is inundated back to the dialysis solution. (DE FRANCISCO, 2000)

2.4 Osmosis (Molecular Water Diffusion)

Osmosis is a diffusion of water through a semipermeable membrane from a solution with a low concentration of the dissolved substance (with high water potential) to the solution with a high concentration of solute (low water potential) in the direction of the solute concentration gradient. The simplest definition is that it is a water diffusion through a semipermeable membrane. (HAYNIE, 2001 s. 130-136)

This is a physical process where the solvent is shifting without energy entering the semipermeable membrane (permeable for the solvent, but impermeable to the dissolved substance), which separates the two solutions from different concentrations. (HARDY, 2003)

Osmosis relaxes energy and can be used to carry out work, as it is in the case of the growing roots of trees broking stones.

This phenomenon is important for the understanding of disequilibrium syndrome.

The main transfer of the solvent takes place from less concentrated (hypotonic) to a more concentrated (hypertonic) solution and tends to reduce the difference in concentrations.

This effect can be added to the increasing pressure of the hypertonic solution in relation to the hypotonic solution.

Osmotic pressure is defined as a colligative trait (Wikipedia. The Free Encyclopedia. Colligative properties, 2009), which means that it depends on the molar concentration of the solution, but not from its type.

Osmosis is important in biological systems, as many biological membranes are semi-permeable. In general, these membranes are weatherproof for organic solutes with large molecules, such as polysaccharides, but water-permeable for small, non-salted solutes. Permeability (throughput) may depend on properties of solubility, electrical properties, or chemistry as well as the size of the solute. Water molecules travel through the plasma membranes of cells, vacuoles or protoplasmic bidirectionally, whether by diffusion through a phospholipid double layer directly or through aquaporins (small transmembrane proteins like those that facilitate diffusion and thereby forming channels). Osmosis provides the primary means by which the water is transported to and from cells. Turgor of the cells is largely maintained by osmosis through the cell membrane between the inside of the cell and its relatively hypotonic environment. (MATON, 1997 s. 66-67)

Osmosis may occur where a partially permeable membrane, such as cell membranes, is present. When the cell is immersed in water, the water molecules pass through the cell membrane from areas with a low concentration of dissolved substances (outside the cell) into an area with a high concentration of solutes (inside the cell). This is called osmosis. The cell membrane is selectively permeable, so the necessary substances can enter the cell, and the waste can be excluded. (MATON, 1997)

When the membrane has the same volume of clean water on both sides, the water molecules pass freely here and there in each direction at the same speed. No main water flow is present on the membrane. However, when the solution is on one side and on the other clean water, the membrane remains to interfere with the molecules on both sides at the same speed. However, some molecules interfering with the membrane from the solution are already molecules of the dissolved substance and do not pass through the membrane. Thus, water molecules pass through the membrane from this side at a lesser frequency. This causes the network flow of water to the solution side. If the membrane is not damaged, this water flow will be slow and eventually stopped as the pressure of the solution on both sides of the reaches the value at which the movement of each direction is the same - a dynamic balance (dynamic adsorption) arises. This may occur since the water potential on both sides of the membrane is the same, or because osmosis is inhibited by factors such as pressure potential or osmotic pressure. (Wikipedia. The Free Encyclopedia. Osmosis, 2009)

Osmosis can also be explained using the terms of entropy from statistical mechanics. As above, it supposes that the permeable membrane separates the same quantities of pure solvent and solution. As the solution has more entropy than a clean solvent, the second thermodynamic law says that the molecules of the solvent will pass into the solution until the entropy of the combined system is maximized. Let us notice that when this happens, the solvent loses entropy until the solution entropy is obtained. Adsorption is balanced; therefore, the maximum entropy is achieved when the gradient entropy drops to zero, and the dissolution occurs. (Wikipedia. The Free Encyclopedia. Osmosis, 2009)

Clean water is more orderly than water in the solution, and therefore, from an entropy point of view, some pure energy moves the water molecule with an unordered solution and "its packing" with clean water. This is the same explanation as to why the unordered air does not spontaneously separate and divide into oxygen and nitrogen. To make this happen energy would be needed. In addition, the particle size does not participate in the osmotic pressure, as it is a fundamental postulate of colligative properties. (BORG, 2003 s. 1-39)

The value of osmotic pressure can be calculated according to classical Van Hoff's formula from 1885

$$\Pi = k.T.c$$
,

Where

- ⇒ Π is osmotic pressure;

- ⇒ **k** is Boltzmann constant (see above in subheading 2.1 Molecular Diffusion);

- ⇒ **T** is the absolute temperature in Kelvin;

- ⇒ **c** is the number of particles of the solute per volume unit, i.e., concentration.

When we imagine that animal plant cell, place it in the sugar or salt water solution, the following cases may occur:

1. The media is **Hypotonic** – A dissolved solution with a higher concentration of water than in the cell – the cell will raise water through osmosis.

2. The media is **Isotonic** – A solution with the same water concentration as in the cell – will not run through the cell membrane.

3. The media is **Hypertonic** – Concentrated solution with a lower water concentration than in cell – the cell will lose water through osmosis.

Osmotic gradient is the difference in concentrations between two solutions to each side of the semipermeable membrane, and it is used to determine the difference in percentage concentration of the specific dissolved particle in the solution.

Usually, the osmotic gradient is used to compare solutions that have a semipermeable membrane that allows water to diffuse between the two solutions towards the hypertonic solution (higher concentration solution). After the water column pressure on the side of the hypertonic solution can compensate for the pressure of water diffusion on the side of the hypotonic solution, thus creating a balance – adsorption. When the balance is reached, it is a dynamic balance. The water is thus still flowing, but the flow rate of both directions was, therefore the solution stabilized-the size of the osmotic pressure on one side and the hydrostatic pressure on the other side was leveled.

2.4.1 Reverse Osmosis

Reverse Osmosis is a filtration process that is used in water treatment. It works by applying pressure to the solution through a membrane that captures the solutes on one side, and, on the other hand, the net solvent-water is switched on. This is a reverse (reversed) process against the normal course of the osmosis process. The pressure used must exceed the osmotic pressure.

The membranes used for reverse osmosis have a dense barrier layer in the polymer matrix, where a larger part of the separation takes place. In most cases, the membrane is designed to allow only water through this dense layer and prevent the passage of dissolved substances (such as salt ions). This process requires high pressure developed on the side with a high concentration of dissolved substances. Usually, its value is achieved in the processing of drinking water from 2 – 17 bars and in the processing of seawater 40 – 70 bars, as this has a natural osmotic pressure of around 24 bars, and it needs to be overcome. (Wikipedia. The Free Encyclopedia. Reverse osmosis, 2009)

The reverse Osmosis is a high-pressure filtration through a very dense membrane. The wide class of undesirable aqueous ingredients is detained by a simple sieve effect as well as electrostatically. Generally, charged particles are detained better than particles electrically neutral and multipower ions better than one-mighty ions. The detention capacity is characterized by the so-called **rejection ratio** that indicates what percentage of the substance is withheld at the water flow by reversed osmosis. This ratio for substances commonly occurring in drinking water ranges from 95% to 99.9%. Microorganisms and endotoxins are reduced at a rate of 1:10 in the passage of water by reversed osmosis. (LOPOT, 2000 s. 112)

To prevent rapid inflammation of the dense membrane the reverse osmosis is usually a certain degree of purity, which is assured in pre-preparatory stages. For the same reason, the flow of its own membrane module is tangential, i.e., the water flows along the membrane and a significant part of the waste. Sometimes this wastewater is referred to as "concentrate" or "retention." (LOPOT, 2000 s. 113)

The ratio of clean water flows to the outlet, the so-called "Permeate," to drain into waste ("concentrate") usually from 2:1 to 1:1. The output flow of clean water is under the same pressure conditions heavily dependent on the water temperature; the decrease in performance with decreasing temperature is 2-3% per 1 °C. Given that the manufacturer usually indicates output flow for the temperature of 15-20°C, it is necessary for the winter period to count about a 1/3 decrease in performance. The capacity of reverse osmosis should, therefore, be chosen with enough reserve. Account should also be taken of the possibility of at least some dialysis devices with a flow of dialysis solution greater than usual 500 mL/min. (LOPOT, 2000 s. 113)

Membrane modules for reverse osmosis have a spiral of guilty leaf membranes. Membrane materials can indicate the acetate cellulose, produced in an asymmetric design with the thin and thick functional layer, that passes to the more powerful supporting structure. Similarly, plastic composite membranes with a thin functional layer of polyamide or polysulfone and a stronger supportive polysulfone structure are constructed. (LOPOT, 2000 s. 113)

Although the reverse osmosis produces high purity water, this water cannot be considered sterile. Regular disinfection of the whole device should be carried out in order to maintain enough microbiological purity of the output water. A usable disinfectant is usually a given membrane material (e.g., polyamide membranes are harmful to chlorine-containing agents). (LOPOT, 2000 s. 113)

The functionality of reverse osmosis can be monitored by measuring the conductivity of the output water. It is indicated in units µS/cm. The tea value is 1 - 5 µS/cm. Under deteriorating effectiveness of reverse osmosis, this value rises. Sometimes a summary of the injection ratio is shown instead of conductivity. The conversion between the two variables is as follows: the reduction ratio (%) = (1-conductivity of the permeation/conductivity of inlet water) x 100. At regular time-outs, it is necessary to carry out microbiological control of the quality of the permeate, both at the exit of the reverse osmosis, as well as at the point of connection of the own dialysis devices. (LOPOT, 2000 s. 113)

3   Hemodialysis, Hemofiltration, and Hemodiafiltration

3.1   Basic Principles

Dialysis is generally a process of the removal of the nitrogenous (and other) waste products of metabolism, and it regulates electrolyte, an aqueous and hepatic acid-base balance associated with renal failure. Dialysis does not regulate endocrine disorders present in renal failure, nor does it prevent cardiovascular complications.

To carry out hemodialysis (HD) a semipermeable membrane should be used to allow the passage of water and solutes with a small molecular weight, but not to pass large molecules (e.g., proteins). In order to have a better idea, an example can be given that the molecular weight of urea is 60 Da (Daltons), creatinine 113 Da, vitamin B_{12} 1355 Da, albumin 60 000 Da and immunoglobulin IgG 140 000 Da. (LEVY, 2004 s. 112)

The extracorporeal circuit of hemodialysis consist of the dialyzer (coil), and a hose system that brings blood to the dialyzer and the purified blood is returned to the patient. With other hoses, the dialysis solution is fed and then drained to the waste. (OPATRNÝ, 2006 s. 386)

Dialysis means diffusion of solutes (dissolved substances in a solution) via a **Semipermeable Membrane** in the direction of the concentration gradient. In the practical implementation of the hemodialysis procedure, other physical and chemical principles an applied such as convection, conduction, adsorption to the surface of the dialysis membrane, and osmosis. (See in more detail Chapter 2 in this work.)

Diffusion is the main mechanism of separation of urea and creatinine and the replacement of serum bicarbonate from the dialysis solution. Diffusion increases proportionally with the size of the concentration difference (concentration gradient) environment (faster movement of molecules) and decreases proportionally with increasing viscosity and the size of the molecules removed. Thus, by increasing the flow of blood and/or dialysis solution, we can achieve an increase in clearance of particularly low molecular weight (urea, creatinine), by maintaining a high concentration gradient and reducing the two components of resistance to diffusion (the stagnant layer of dialysis solution and the stagnant layer of blood). The characteristics of the membrane also affect the speed of diffusion. For example, high-flux membranes are thin and have large pores, and in such a way, they achieve low resistance to diffusion. Protein-bound substances are not removed by the dialysis by diffusion, as proteins do not pass through the dialysis membrane, only the free (unbound) fraction of these substances are removed.

The term ultrafiltration (UF) means the filtrated water with the dissolved solutes in the direction of the pressure gradient, which is caused by hydrostatic or osmotic forces (See above in Chapter 2). During hemodialysis, ultrafiltration is usually achieved by the negative pressure generated on the side of the dialysis compartment by means of a drainage pump (transmembrane pressure, "TMP"). The rate of ultrafiltration depends on the pressure gradient. The dialysis membranes differed with their permeability for water and based on which we divide them into "high-flux" and "low-flux" membranes. The permeability of the membrane is expressed as the ultrafiltration filter coefficient KU_f in mL/hour/mmHg and usually ranges between 2 and 50 mL/hour/mmHg. Central water permeability membranes have KU_f ranging from 5 to 10 mL/hour/mmHg and membranes with a value of KU_f above 10 mL/hour/mmHg is indicated as a membrane with high aqueous permeability. (LEVY, 2004 s. 112)

Diafiltrating is the concomitant use of dialysis and ultrafiltration in order to achieve clearance of solutes and water. Filtration is a process identical to the process described as ultrafiltration, but as opposed to ultrafiltration, the volume of the removed filtrate is replaced by the replacement (substitution) solution in the elimination methods using hemofiltration. Therefore, ultrafiltration is called the volume of the filtrate, which is not a substitute for substitution and allows, inter alia, the achievement of negative fluid balances during the extra-body (extracorporeal) elimination procedure.

Simply, the dialysis device or machine (dialysis monitor) pumps the blood, and the dialysis solution in the opposite course through the dialyzer (coil). However, the hemodialysis device is a complex device and contains a large number of safety feature, pump drivers, pressure and flow sensors and monitors, air leakage detectors, mechanisms to change the composition of dialysis solution, blood pressure monitors, and even systems for monitoring biochemical parameters of blood, monitoring of blood flow in the vascular access, monitoring of the delivered dialysis dose and devices allowing remote control, control and transmission of data to the remote databases.

Dialysis solution is a solution composed of purified water, sodium, potassium, magnesium, calcium, chlorides, bicarbonate and/or acetate or citrate and possibly glucose. Blood and dialysis solution are separated by the semipermeable membrane in the dialyzer. Since dialysis solution does not contain any waste products of metabolism (urea, creatinine, etc.), these substances are dispatched from the blood to dialysis solution. The diffusion is maximized by maintaining high blood flow and dialysis solution and by pumping two solutions (blood and dialysis solution) in opposite directions (counter flow). The conjunctions clearance may be supplemented by the formation of transmembrane pressure in the dialysis solution. To avoid penetration of dialysis solution into the blood, we try to set the TMP to reach the UF at 100 – 200 mL/hr.

This procedure is well for the removal of the low-molecular substances, but it is not enough to remove medium molecular toxins and phosphates. This led to the development of other related methods such as hemodiafiltration, with high volumes of ultrafiltrate replaced by a substitution (replacement) solution, thereby ensuring improved clearance of medium molecules and phosphates.

Caution should be exercised during the first hemodialysis procedure of the patient in order to avoid disequilibrium syndrome. The parameters of the procedure must be adjusted so as not to reduce the concentration of the urea by more than 30%, i.e., by about one third. Its length is typically within 2 hours, and the blood flow is 150 – 200 mL/min and the use of high-permeable dialyzer is usually inappropriate.

A tactic of chronic dialysis therapy such as the frequency of dialysis depends on the metabolic and nutritional condition of the patient. If the residual diuresis is greater than 1500 mL per 24 hours, the patient should have prescribed the HD 2 x 5 hours a week, at a lower diuresis it is 3 x 4 hours per week. (MYDLÍK, 2004 s. 753) However, the European guidelines for good practice EBPG currently recommend a standard dose of dialysis 3 x 4 hours per week for all patients. The same it is in KDIGO and K/DOQI guidelines and US NKF recommendations.

3.2 Factors affecting the clearance of the solutes

Clearance is a measure of the amount of blood "purified" of a given salt and measured in mL/min. Dialysis reduces the concentration of waste solutes during the blood passage, and this can be best measured by clearance. Five basic factors may be established when considering the magnitude of the clearance of individual solutes.

1. **The blood flow rate.**

   The rate of blood flow is usually maintained at a level of 200 – 500 mL/min. Increasing the rate of blood flow increases the clearance of the solutes, but this increase in clearance is not proportional to the increase in blood flow rate. The efficiency of diffusion is reduced with rising blood flow rates. Generally, a 100% increase in blood flow rates can achieve the 20 – 50% increase of urea clearance (LEVY, 2004 s. 116). It is even less effective for the solutes with a larger molecular weight (middle molecular weight catabolites).

2. **The flow rate of the dialysis solution.**

Normally, the speed of the dialysis solution flow rate is approximately 500 mL/min. The most recent feature is the use of the factor that multiple blood flow, thus gaining the value of the dialysis solution flow, so for example, at a blood flow rate of 300 mL/min and a commonly used factor of 1.5, dialysis solution will run at a speed of 450 mL/min.

Increasing the flow rate of dialysis solution increases the clearance of the solutes, but unfortunately only marginally. When the flow rate of the dialysis solution is increased from 500 to 800 mL/min, more than 10% of urea clearance is achieved (LEVY, 2004 s. 116). However, it should be noted that the clearance achieved in practice is slightly higher than those found in vitro.

3. **The efficacy of the dialysis.**

For the clearance of the solutes, the membrane thickness, pore size, and the architecture and geometry of the dialyzer are important. The efficacy of the clearance of solutes is expressed by CoA (Mass Transfer Urea Coefficient), and the manufacturers indicate this for each dialyzer. Most dialyzers have a CoA or KoA of approximately 300 – 500. In the case of high-efficacy dialyzers (High-Efficiency Dialyzers), this value increases up to 700. The change to high-efficiency dialysis has the most significant effect on increasing the urea clearance, opposed to the weak effect of increasing the blood flow rate or the flow of dialysis solution (LEVY, 2004 s. 116)

4. **The molecular weight of the solute.**

Larger molecules and therefore substances with the larger molecular weight, are removed slowly and therefore have reduced clearances. Increasing blood flow has a minor effect on increasing clearance of substances with large or middle molecular weight than in substances with a smaller molecular weight.

5. **Time.**

Length (time duration) of the procedure/treatment is one of the most important determinants of the magnitude of the clearance of the solutes and thus the effectiveness of their removal from the patient's body. Changes to other parameters of the hemodialysis procedure are carried out mostly to shorten the time duration of this procedure and thus shorten the time that the patient must spend on dialysis. This is based on the requirements of patients. Enough clearance of low molecular weight solutes can usually be achieved even during shorter hemodialysis using "high-flux" membranes, increased blood flow and the like, but the long-term results of such a procedure remain still unclear, especially when we speak about the control of the extracellular volume and clearance of larger molecules. The extracellular volume control remains largely inadequate, interdialytic weight gain often exceeds an acceptable value of 2-3% or even 4-5% of the so-called patient's dry body weight, resulting in the persistence of hypertension and the lack of elimination of solutes with greater molecular weight and phosphates with their implications for chronic complications of long-term hemodialysis therapy (increases cardiovascular morbidity and mortality, highlights and accelerates renal osteodystrophy etc.).

3.3 Ultrafiltration during hemodialysis

During the hemodialysis procedure, ultrafiltration can remove water with substances in the water dissolved, which are removed by convection (membrane filtration). Terminologically it is true to say that ultrafiltration eliminates fluid, not just water itself.

Ultrafiltration during conventional hemodialysis is used simply for removal of excessively accumulated water between hemodialysis treatments due to food, fluid, and metabolic water, and thus allows us to balance the intake and supply of fluids in a given patient and to excrete accumulated water, due to the limited or completely absent kidney capacity of the urination in these patients. After Counting the estimated amount of water breathing, faeces and sweat (insensible perspiration) normally and deducing them water metabolic rate, we are at a value of about 650 mL, which, together with the volume of diuresis in a given patient, becomes a retro-reflector for us to calculate the authorized fluid intake so that the patient does not exceed the interdialytic mass increment at 2-3% of its 'dry' body weight.

Ultrafiltration is achieved by creating the transmembrane gradient in the dialyzer. In older devices intended for the implementation of hemodialysis, the transmembrane pressure (TMP) is directly measured, and the required UF is achieved by manipulating the TMP value. The most advanced instruments use a volumetric control that continuously directly measure the passing and leaking volumes of the dialyzer, and the amount of ultrafiltration is determined from their difference. Thus, as regards the methods of ultrafiltration during hemodialysis, we distinguish the pressure and volumetric control of ultrafiltration.

1. *Pressure control of ultrafiltration.*

The pressure in the blood compartment of the dialyzer is usually + 50 to + 100 mmHg depending on the blood flow rate but may be higher during venous stenosis. The pressure in the dialyzer compartment can be reduced by limiting the flow rate of the dialysis solution when the pump reduces the outflow from the dialyzer. In this way, negative pressure can be achieved in the value of 500 mmHg. However, greater pressure may lead to dialyzer rupture. Pressures are usually measured on the blood output and the output of dialyzer, so be aware that the dialyzer itself is about something above and, finally, that some devices measure the pressure on the inlet.

The transmembrane pressure (TMP) needed to remove a given fluid volume can be calculated based on the ultrafiltration coefficient of the dialyzer (KU_f), the value of which is provided by its manufacturer. However, most of the devices are constructed by automatically calculating the necessary TMP to achieve the required UF.

2. *Volumetric control of ultrafiltration.*

This method of controlling ultrafiltration is more accurate, that is particularly important when using higher flow membranes ("high-flux" membranes). Small errors in the measurement of TMP (in the pressure control method of ultrafiltration) can cause large volume changes. In addition, the ultrafiltration coefficient (CU_f) of the dialyzer in the hemodialysis procedure should be altered as a result of increased protein deposition, partial blood clotting, and hematocrit changes. Systems with volumetric control measure the maturity of ultrafiltration directly, and by quantification of the volume of dialyzer through the dialyzer, and therefore not susceptible to such problems.

To achieve adequate clearance of the solutes by filtration, it is necessary to remove the large volumes of liquid, resulting in the need for substitution/replacement of these volumes to the patient, and thus the need for highly purified water or replacement (substitution) solutions, as these need to be in large volume injected to the patient. However, ultrafiltration provides better clearance of solutes with a large molecular weight (e.g., β2-Microglobulin) by convection and is associated with greater cardiovascular stability than conventional hemodialysis. These procedures shall apply to the implementation of hemofiltration, hemodiafiltration, and related methods.

3.4 High-Efficiency and "High-Flux" Hemodialysis

3.4.1 Highly effective (high efficacy) hemodialysis ("High-Efficiency Dialysis")

High-efficiency hemodialysis is defined by a high *Clearance of Urea* that is greater than **210 mL/min** and high CoA urea (Mass Transfer Coefficient x Surface Area), which is greater than **600 mL/min**. Ultrafiltration coefficient KU_f may be low or high, and cellulose or synthetic membrane is used. It is important to note that at low blood flow with rates below 200 mL/min, creatinine clearance is the same as for regular "low-efficiency" dialysis. The higher flow of the dialysis solution (more than 500 mL/min) increases the clearance of the solutes only at blood flow higher than 200 mL/min. Hemodialysis with high efficacy (high-efficiency hemodialysis) requires membrane with the large surface, high CoA, high levels of blood flow rate and the high flow of dialysate and bicarbonate hemodialysis (not acetate). It also requires excellent vascular access, which provides adequate blood flow (not standard percutaneous catheters).

3.4.2 „High-Flux" Hemodialysis

The term "high-flux" dialysis refers to the speed of transport of the water through the dialysis membrane and is usually synonymous with the use of a highly permeable membrane with the clearance of β2-Microglobulin greater than 20 mL/min. Such dialysis requires a volumetric control of ultrafiltration to avoid catastrophic water depletion. Clearance of substances with medium and large molecular weight is better due to the greater size of pores in the membrane. Dialyzer can be synthetic or cellulose-free. The necessity is the ultrapure dialysis solution and the use of bicarbonate due to the risk of retrospective filtration from the dialysis solution to the blood.

Some evidence from short-term clinical trials (mostly with a small number of patients and not prospective one) indicate that "high-flux" dialyzers with biocompatible membranes may lead to better maintenance of the residual renal function, less inflammatory response, higher albumin serum levels, a better nutritional condition, less dyslipidemia, lower levels of β2-Microglobulin and minor dialysis amyloidosis. A large randomized, Hemo prospective study showed no benefit of a "high-flux" membrane as for morbidity or mortality. (LEVY, 2004 s. 122)

3.5 Hemofiltration and Hemodiafiltration

Hemofiltration provides the clearance of the solutes exclusively by convection when the dissolved substances are navigated together with the solvent flow through the semipermeable membrane in the direction of the effective pressure gradient. This eliminates relatively high volumes of filtrate (> 40 liters in a single procedure), which are replaced by a replacement (substitution) solution.

Hemodiafiltration combines hemodialysis with higher ultrafiltration volumes than for hemofiltration, i.e., combines convectional as well as diffuse removal of renal retention solutes and other substances from the blood that passes through the semi-permeable dialysis membrane. (EISELT, 2002)

The replacement fluid (substitution solution) must be ultrapure, with minimal contamination of the endotoxins because it is administered directly to the patient's blood. A high permeable membrane, high blood flow and precise control of the volume of the replacement solution are also needed.

Hemofiltration provides better removal of substances with the larger relative molecular weight (for example β_2-Microglobulin, end glucose degradation products, etc.), improved clearance of uremic toxins with a low relative molecular weight and improved cardiovascular stability and control of blood pressure versus traditional intermittent hemodialysis. They also improve the markers of inflammation. It is particularly beneficial for patients who are treated with dialysis for the very long time without the prospect of a possible renal transplantation treatment, or for patients with a high weight and/or height, for whom an adequate Kt/V value cannot be achieved with normal hemodialysis. In hemofiltration and hemodiafiltration, there is a lower incidence of intradialytic complications. For these techniques, short-term studies have shown higher serum albumin levels and higher hemoglobin levels, decreased the incidence of pruritus, reduced ESA need, increased Kt/V values, reduced need for a surgical procedure for decompression in the carpal tunnel, reduced need for phosphate binders, improved nutrient indices and possible reduction of mortality. (LEVY, 2004 s. 124)

Historically, these are financially significantly more demanding procedures compared to conventional hemodialysis, but the economic difference was significantly reduced after the introduction of the continuous production of clean replacement solutions from dialysis concentrates ("online" HF, HDF), powdered alkaline concentrates (BiCart or BiBag) and after introduction water filtration by additional two or three special filters in newer dialysis monitors. In such cases, the volume of ultrafiltration varies at 60 - 90 liter per week and 9 – 15 liters to one HDF procedure with the aim of more than 23 liters for one postdilution "online" HDF treatment.

Hemodiafiltration has several modifications. These include:

1. Non-Acetate Biofiltration (**AFB** – Acetate Free Biofiltration).

2. Dialysis with Paired Filtration (**PFD** – Paired Filtration Dialysis).

AFB, PFD, and their modifications are undoubtedly effective methods of blood purification. But whether they are more beneficial than normal hemodiafiltration, is still very questionable and not scientifically proven. Rather, it seems that for the success of hemodiafiltration therapy is more important the volume of the filtrate than the modification characterizing AFB or PFD. A multicenter clinical trial is needed to give evidence of the status of the above RRT methods. (TESAŘ, 2006 s. 516)

3.5.1 Acetate Free Biofiltration (AFB)

In acetate-free biofiltration, a dialysis solution is free of any acetate. The bicarbonate is infused to the venous distribution of the extracorporeal (extra-body) circuit. The authors of the method are confident that even a small quantity of acetate in dialysate represents a disadvantage in compensation of metabolic acidosis and can cause adverse reactions. In particular, the reduced contractility, possible infarction, oxidative and carbonyl stress are mentioned. In some studies, AFB has improved renal anemia compared to bicarbonate hemodialysis. However, it is not yet explained whether this is specifically due to AFB. In this was at AFB compared to the bicarbonate dialysis used a pass-through membrane, the membranes were made from different material, and the treatment dose according to Kt/V was higher for AFB.

3.5.2 Paired Filtration Dialysis (PFD)

For Paired Filtration Dialysis a device is used where one part forms a filter with a high permeable membrane and second dialyzer with a low permeable dialysis membrane. In the first part, the blood is cleaned by filtration and in the second by diffusion. Both processes are separate, and there is no interference. Some studies argue that in the PFD compared to conventional hemodiafiltration, the development of proinflammatory cytokine IL-1 is higher and that patients have lower plasma concentrations of C-reactive protein and interleukin 1 (PANICHI, 1998).

3.5.3 *HFR Online*

A newer modification of PFD is the HFR online (Hemodiafiltration with On-Line Endogenous Reinfusion). In the filter, the resulting filtrate is cleaned by passing through the adsorber and reinfused to the next part of the device that is the dialyzer. Cleansing and Adsorbing are removed for the blood, creatinine, urea, B2M (β2-Microglobulin) and other substances. By using a blood filtrate as replacement fluid, some important substances such as hormones, amino acids or vitamins are returned to the body. (TESAŘ, 2006 s. 516)

3.6 Dialysis Membranes

The development of the membrane has its roots in the textile industry. Currently, dialysis membranes are only produced in 4 countries of the world: France, Japan, Germany, and the USA. The largest suppliers in Europe are Akzo, Fresenius, Gambro B. Braun, and Hospal (a subsidiary of Gambro). In Japan, they are manufactured by Asahi, Kuraray, Kawasaki, Nikkiso, Terumo, Teijin, Toray, and Toyobo. V The US there is the sole producer of Althin (CD-Medical), Minntech and National Medical Care (NMC). (KADLEC, 1997 s. 183)

The classic dialysis membranes are divided into two groups:

1. Cellulose-based dialysis membranes.

2. Synthetic Polymers Dialysis Membranes.

Newer types of membranes are also developed; for example, the membrane surface is bound by vitamin E and so on.

3.6.1 Cellulose-based dialysis membranes

Cellulose membranes can cause complement and leucocytes to be activated, while synthetic membranes are characterized by higher biocompatibility in this respect. The unmodified cellulose membranes are low-flow low-permeable (low-flux). Modified cellulose membranes can be as low-flow and high-flow, high-permeable (high-flux) with higher (triacetate cellulose) or lower (acetate cellulose) biocompatibility. **Cellulose-based** dialysis membranes include:

a. Dialysis membranes from **Unmodified Cellulose**, e.g., Cellulose Type FIN (Cuprophan® Akzo, Bioflux® Akzo – Cuprammonium Rayon, Cuprammonium Boiler

b. Dialysis membranes from **Regenerated Cellulose**, e.g., the membrane of the company Asahi

c. **Synthetically modified** membranes with the chemical modification of the whole basis. The whole basis consists of 2 molecules of glucose bound in 1,4-beta-glucananic configurations. The glucose molecule contains 3 OH (hydroxy) groups that react easily, namely:

a) Esterification with DEAE-groups (Hemophan® + DEAE Akzo), benzyl groups (SMC + Benzyl Akzo) or by replacing with the polyethylene glycol (PEG-RC) chain

b) Esterification of acetyl groups. The dialysis membranes of the saponified cellulose ester – *cellulose acetate dialysis membranes*, e.g., cellulose-acetate dialysis membrane of Althin and Toyobo, cellulose-acetate dialysis membrane of Akzo and Althin, and cellulose triacetate dialysis membrane of Althin and Toyobo

c) Surface packaging of a synthetic polymer. These are dialysis membranes with the so-called coating of Asahi, polyethylene glycol cellulose, and of the company Asahi). (KADLEC, 1997 s. 183)

3.6.2 Dialysis membranes with synthetic polymers

The second large group of dialysis membranes is formed by the dialysis membranes made of the synthetic polymers. In their use, a higher clearance of β2-Microglobulin compared to cellulose membranes at the equal clearance of the solutes is achieved (LEVY, 2004 s. 130). They are obtained by different methods of hydrophilization. This includes polysulfone, polyacrylonitrile, and polyamide. They are hydrophobic and must, therefore, be adapted to hydrophilic ones to be used as a filter for toxins in the blood, e.g., by hydrophilic *ethyl vinyl copolymers*, so they can be used without modification. Biocompatibilities efficacy of dialysis membranes depends on the consequences of the two processes induced by hydrophilization:

1. *Complement activation* observed in polysulfone membranes, which depend on certain hydrophilic additives such as polyvinyl pyrrolidone

2. *The formation of bradykinin* in polyacrylonitrile membranes, which depends on the ingredients used for their copolymerization

Hydrophilization is used in different methods. Polymers are mixed with hydrophilic agents, such as polyethylene glycol, polyvinyl pyrrolidone, and others, or copolymerized with hydrophilic polymers, such as acrylamide or methyl sulfonate. The third option of hydrophilization is the adjustment during the extrusion of the membrane capillaries (helixone – nanotechnological treatment of the pores of the polysulfone membrane).

The dialysis membranes of synthetic polymers include:

1. ***Polyacrylonitrile membranes*** (**PAN**, *Funck-Brentano et all, 1972*) – AN 69® Hospal, PAN-DX® Asahi, SPAN® Akzo

2. ***Polysulfone membranes*** (**PSU**, *Streicher and Streicher, 1985; Schäfer et all., 1989*) – PS400® Fresenius, SPE® Akzo, F6/F60® Fresenius, PS-K® Kuraray, Polyphen® Minntech, Biosulfane® NMC, Pepa® Nikkiso

3. ***Polyamide membranes*** (**PA**, *Deppisch et all, 1992*) – Poryflux® Gambro, FH 88®

4. ***Membranes of ethyl vinyl copolymers*** (**Eval**) – Eval C® Kuraray, Eval D®

5. ***Polycarbonate membranes*** (*Göhl et all, 1986*) – Polycarbonate® Gambro

6. ***Polyester blend membranes*** - Polyacrylics + polyether sulfonate (*Shimizu et all., 1992*) – Pepa® Nikkiso

For hemofiltration (continuous or high flow) and in related methods, only synthetic membranes are used.

There are also data suggesting the use of the membranes covered by vitamin E (e.g., **excebrane**) to reduce the formation of free oxygen radicals, thereby achieving higher biocompatibility. Furthermore, a membrane of AN69 was prepared using the binding of polyethyleneimine (**AN69ST**), which binds heparin and allows a substantial reduction in the dose of heparin needed to prevent precipitation in the extracorporeal circuit - it is usually enough to give the heparin prior to the beginning of the procedure. (LEVY, 2004 s. 130)

3.6.3 Reactions to dialysis membranes

These reactions do not, in any case, be a reaction to the membrane itself but maybe a reaction to the substance used to sterilize the dialyzer, some other medicine, the activation of the complement or unknown mechanisms. Sometimes these reactions are called reactions of the first use of dialyzer ("first use reactions"), but they also occur with the repeated use of dialyzers. These reactions can be divided into two types:

A. The reaction type of "A"

They appear within minutes after the initiation of the dialysis and are manifested by shortness of breath, wheezing, feeling of warmth, hives, coughs, hypotension, collapse or in the worst case of cardiac arrest. Predominantly due to an immune response to ethylene oxide, and they occur in patients who are taking ACE inhibitors and use dialysis membrane AN69 (or rarely used by other types of PAN membranes). However, the fact that the AN69 membrane can increase the levels of bradykinin should also be noted in patients who are not taking ACE inhibitors.

B. The reaction type of "B"

This type of reaction is much more common, but their progress is also much milder. They usually appear 20 – 40 minutes after the initiation of the dialysis procedure and are manifested by back pain or chest pain. The cause is still unknown.

Other reactions to dialysis membranes are also rarely described. In 1990, patients were reported with acute deafness syndrome and blindness after the treatment with the old dialyzers with the cellulose membrane over 11 years old. None of these patients were healed, and all died within 1 year. In 2002, many patients died after using dialyzer with a cellulose-acetate membrane in Baxter's dialyzer, called Althane. The cause of death was residual perfluorocarbon located in dialyzers. It is a volatile hydrophobic fluid completely insoluble in water, which led to massive gas formation on the right side of the heart and the blockade of pulmonary capillaries. Perfluorocarbon was used to repair insoluble hollow fibers during the manufacture of a dialyzer. (LEVY, 2004 s. 132)

3.6.4 Biocompatibility of Dialysis Membranes

Dialysis membranes may have and have different effects on cells and proteins that are exposed to them. As biocompatible, we can consider the membrane that produces the least inflammatory response in patients exposed to it, i.e., it does not cause the activation of the complement, and cell activation and minimum interaction with proteins and are not thrombogenic (causing low thrombin formation and platelet release factor 4). (LEVY, 2004 s. 134) The biocompatibility of the dialyzer affects its design, geometry, and architecture as well as the nature of the dialysis membrane. Hydroxyl groups on the surface of the unmodified cellulose are activated by an alternative route of complement and subsequently cells a destructed. Substituted cellulose and synthetic membranes cause in general less activation of the complement, but also strongly bind the proteins of the complement and prevent retrograde penetration into circulation.

As has been said in contact with a dialysis membrane, the complement is activated by an alternative route but also the formation of anaphylatoxin, in contact with the coagulation system activate factor XII and the internal route of activation of the hemocoagulation cascade, an increase in serum levels of certain cytokines, rarely to hemolysis; neutrophils react with leukopenia, increased excretion of adhesion molecules, degranulation, and release of free oxygen radicals, lymphocytes are activated, but there is damage to the proliferation of T-cells, a decreased response of monocytes and increased (interleukin-1) and platelet activation, increased adhesion, and subsequently thrombocytopenia and platelet aggregation 4 and ADP are activated. (LEVY, 2004 s. 134)

Improved biocompatibility is associated with the following positive consequences:

- Decreased deposition of amyloid

- Uncommon hypersensitivity reactions

- Decreased incidence of intradialytic hypotension

- Slower loss of residual renal function after starting the chronic intermittent hemodialysis program

- Decreased incidence of infections

- Improved nutritional status

- Reduced catabolism of proteins

- Improved lipid profiles

- Possible improved long-term morbidity and mortality

Unfortunately, in some cases data contradict each other, the results of studies comparing dialyzers and the clinical significance of increased biocompatibility remain controversial. But it should be noted that current European Directives (EBPG = European Best Practice Guidelines) recommend greater pores, high throughput and increased biocompatibility of membranes, which can be considered as binding. The same is in KDIGO, K/DOQI and US NKF recommendations.

3.7 Dialyzers

Dialyzer (also called a filter or coil) consists of a rigid capsule usually produced from polyurethane, in which hollow fibers are placed, i.e., capillaries or parallel plates made from the dialysis membrane. It also has two inputs to inflow and drains the blood and two additional inputs to circulate the dialysis solution. Capillary or parallel plates allow the area of the dialysis membrane to be maximized, that maximizes blood and dialysis solution contact. In the compilation of newer dialyzer, other techniques, as well as nanotechnologies for the arrangement of capillaries in the dialyzer, are also applied, so that the effectiveness of the contact surface of the membrane with blood and dialysis solution increased further. When capillaries for dialysate and the blood (interior capillaries) passes alternately between the different layers of the dialysis membrane.

Capillary dialyzers have a slightly smaller filling volume and may be easier to retain ethylene oxide (if used as a sterilization agent), while for plates dialyzer the benefit is less risk of blood clotting in the dialyzer. At present, the capillary dialyzer is most commonly used in all countries because of their higher efficiency.

Thinking about ideal dialyzer, we could postulate several criteria that should be met by such dialyzer. participation, it must be held that There is currently no dialyzer that perfectly meets all these criteria. These are:

1. High clearance of toxins with a small and medium relative molecular weight

2. Adequate ultrafiltration

3. Negligible loss of protein and amino acids

4. Non-toxic composition

5. Minimum activation of blood clotting cells and pathways

6. Minimum blood filling volume.

7. Reliability

8. The possibility of re-use (unlike in the USA, in Slovakia an many other countries the reuse of dialyzer is not allowed by legislation, it is prohibited)

9. Low price

In general, the technical specifications for commonly used dialyzers are as follows:

> The filling volumes range from 40 to 150 mL (do not include blood volume in dialysis-tubes, which represents approximately 150 mL).

> The membrane surface ranges from 0.5 to 2.2 m^2.

> U_f is from 2.5 to 85 mL/h/mmHg. Cellulose membranes (and most of the modified cellulose membranes) have $U_f < 10$. For the < 4 goes on throughput and > 8 on high throughput. A membrane with high permeability requires a

dialysis monitor with a volumetric control of ultrafiltration due to safety.

- The CoA ranges from 200 to 1200 (< 300 represents low-efficiency dialyzer, > 600 dialyzes with high efficiency).

- In the package leaflets, the clearance values for urea and vitamin B may still be found, sometimes for creatinine, phosphates, and inulin, in blood flow ranging from 200 to 400 mL/min, as well as the conversion coefficients for albumin (should be zero) and β_2-Microglobulin.

- The dialyzer is sterilized by gamma-rays, ethylene oxide or water steam. Water vapor and radiation represent the lowest risk to the patients, like ethylene oxide, must be thoroughly rinsed prior to the use of the dialyzer.

- Dialyzer should be flushed before use with > 2 liters of the flushing solution before it is attached to the patient to prevent the release of fragments from the dialysis circuit and to remove other potential contaminants or residues from the production of sterilization substances.

3.8 Dialysis device (machine, monitor)

Dialysis devices, sometimes also called dialysis monitors, basically consist of several basic parts.

1. *Blood pump*. Usually, peristaltic blood pumps with blood flow used during the procedure of 200 – 600 mL/min.

2. *Air detector*. It minimalizes the risk of the air embolism and prevents the detection of airborne distally in the venous balloon of venous dialysis bring the air to the patient's return on blood. This is usually an ultrasound detection. It is connected to the flap, which immediately stops the blood flow to the patient in case of air detection.

3. *Heparin administration system*. Usually in the form of an integrated injector on the syringe.

4. *A system for the preparation of dialysis*. The latter blends in a proportion that is given to the one-which type of apparatus, three components: water, acidic and alkaline concentrate. In some devices, this part may be absent, where the central preparation and the delivery of dialysis are used. Acidic concentrates are usually acetate

(the concentration of acetate depends on the type of the dialyzer) and liquid. Alkaline concentrates constituting bicarbonate may be liquid, or a powder form of sodium hydrogen carbonate in a bag or capsule, from which a saturated solution is prepared during the procedure in the apparatus. The dialyzer gets rid of dissolved gases and heats to the temperature of 35.5°C to a maximum of 38°C according to the current setting of the device. The dialysis pump also allows the formation of negative pressure on the side of the dialyzer in dialysis for the purpose of achieving the desired ultrafiltration. It includes temperature and conductivity monitoring.

5. *Control of Ultrafiltration.* Typically, volumetric control of ultrafiltration is used through flow sensors on the inlet and exit of the dialyzer. The pressure control is not used because of its lack of accuracy. TMP is adjusted to achieve the required rate of ultrafiltration. Pressure can be achieved in the volumetric control of UF and is at about ± 0.5% (approx. 25 mL/h) and can be programmed to vary the speed of UF during the procedure, what is called **Sequential Ultrafiltration**, or you can use **ultrafiltration profiling**. The maximum speed of UF is

approximately 4 liters. Non-Disciplined patients with high interdialytic weight increases and there is sometimes a need to use higher levels.

6. *Profiling of sodium.* Most devices allow you to adjust the sodium level in dialysis solution and at the same time adjust this setting during dialysis either manually or by preprogramming a certain profile of the sodium concentration.

7. *Additional Ultrafiltrate* and/or dialysis solution. These allow you to use the so-called "online" hemofiltration and hemodiafiltration preparation of ultrafiltrate dialysis, which is a condition for the use of high-permeable membranes due to the possibility of backward filtration.

8. *Automatic chemical and thermal disinfection.* This can be pre-programmed or performed manually.

9. *Dialysis with one needle (called Single-Needle Dialysis, in a nutshell, S/N HD) or two needles (standard, so-called Double-needle dialysis, an abbreviation is D/N HD).* Each device already usually allows you to use both options. S/N HD requires only one functional needle, but it is less

effective and increases the risk and value of recirculation. It is used in the Y-connector. It can be done by system pressure-Pressure or even a time-time system. Some systems also enable so-called cross-over single needle HD (B. Braun).

10. *Pressure detectors.* They are usually placed in front of a blood buffer, sometimes a blood pump and dialyzer. In some cases, an open pressure detector is also present in the dialyzer compartment. The arterial detector monitors pressure fluctuations due to blood flow problems by the dialysis access. The venous detector picks the pressure differences due to the rise of resistance on the side of the venous return. Both detectors are connected to alarms and blood flow in the extracorporeal circuit. The last detector is the transmembrane pressure detector (TMP). It indicates the current hydrostatic gradient on the membrane.

11. *The detector of blood leakage.* It monitors whether dialyzer has not been rupturing by infrared radiation and photodetector by monitoring the eventual presence of blood in dialyzer leaving the dialyzer. Sensitivity is < 0.5 mL of blood per minute.

12. *The detector of blood present in extracorporeal circulation.* It is usually located between the air detector and the throttle of the Extracorporeal (Extra-Body) circulation.

13. More modern devices also include special monitors for the calculation and monitoring of the Kt/V value in real time, automatic monitoring of blood pressure and/or ECG, modules monitoring blood volume (prevention of intradialytic hypotension by monitoring hematocrit or protein concentrations of optical or ultrasonic sensors), monitors current oxygen saturation, monitor balance fluids and hydration of the patient (measured by the plasma refilling ratio), measurement of recirculation, etc.

3.9 Dialysis solutions

Dialysis solutions are usually prepared from concentrates and the buffer system (puffer) containing either acetate or bicarbonate or citrate. Acetate alone is currently very rarely used, mostly in developing countries. The exact composition can be adjusted as needed, and the use of the individualized composition of the dialysis solution is increased for the patient, which brings increased requirements for the logistics of the dialysis centers. Modern dialysis devices already allow the precise preparation of the dialysis solution and the monitoring of its composition by measuring conductivity. The second option is the central preparation of dialysis solution from concentrates in the dialysis center and the transferring of the pre-finished dialysis solutions to individual dialysis devices. But central preparation does not allow individualization of dialysis solutions for individual patients.

Another method is to provide the dialysis solution in so-called batches. The known system is, e.g., Genius by Fresenius.

In the past, acetate dialysis was very widely used since only one concentrate containing all components of the dialysis solution was used, making it easier for production. Later, the concentrates were given with a bicarbonate content, and instead of the so-called of acetal dialysis, bicarbonate dialysis was introduced. This is more appropriate and allows to induce fewer complications and side effects during dialysis. In some cases, the citrate is possible to be used instead of the acetate. However, during production and storage, there is precipitation bicarbonate. Therefore magnesia and calcium have been added to bicarbonate to prevent the precipitation of carbonate crystals. The dialysis solution can also be prepared by mixing three components: electrolytes and glucose + sodium chloride + bicarbonate. This will achieve a finer adjustment of the individual components of the solution.

The usual composition of dialysate (dialysis solution) is as follows:

Sodium (Natrium)	132 – 155	mmol/L
Potassium (Kalium)	0 – 4	mmol/L
Calcium	1 – 2	mmol/L
Magnesium (Magnesia)	0.5 – 1	mmol/L
Chlorides	90 – 120	mmol/L
Acetate	30 – 45	mmol/L (only in acetate dialysis)
Bicarbonate	27 – 40	mmol/L
Glucose (dextrose)	0 – 5.5	mmol/L
pH	7.1 – 7.3	

Sometimes the composition of the dialysis solution is indicated separately for the dialysis solution for acetoacetate and bicarbonate dialysis as follows (TESAŘ, 2006 s. 531):

	Bicarbonate Dialysis Solution	Acetate Dialysis Solution
Sodium (Na)	**137 – 144**	**132 – 145**
Potassium (K)	**0 – 4**	**0 – 4**

Calcium (Ca)	1.25 – 2	1.5 – 2
Magnesium (Mg)	0.25 – 1	0.5 – 1
Chlorides (CL)	98 – 112	99 – 110
Acetate	2.5 – 10	31 – 45
Bicarbonate (NaHCO3)	27 – 38	0
Glucose	0 – 11	0 – 11

Numerical values are given in units of [mmol/L].

Lower sodium levels in the solution are used to minimize hypertension. However, the complication is a high incidence of convulsions and disequilibrium symptoms, hypotension, and hypertension induced by the renin-angiotensin system stimulation. Higher sodium concentrations are used to minimize muscle spasms, nausea, vomiting, and hypotension. Concentrations are used up to 150 mmol/L. However, higher levels of sodium in the dialysis solution may increase thirst and induce hypertension in the long-term view for the accumulation of salt and water. The disadvantages can be compensated by the profiling of sodium levels in the dialysis solution during the dialysis procedure. In the introduction, higher levels of sodium are used in the solution, which gradually decreases during the dialysis procedure according to different schemes (depending on the software of the dialysis device), in order to achieve a balanced sodium balance according to the baseline sodium levels.

In patients with repeated vomiting and diarrhea, higher levels of potassium in the dialysis solution are sometimes required. These should always be determined according to the patient's current clinical condition. Potassium levels of 2 or 3 mmol/L are commonly used and usually no need to be altered in stable patients.

A certain level (equivalent to the level of ionized calcium) is necessary to prevent hypocalcemia during the hemodialysis procedure. Dialysis solutions with low calcium levels (1.25 mmol/L) are required in patients with uncontrolled hyperparathyroidism and hypercalcemia. When using citrate acid concentrate, it is not recommended to use the low-calcium solution due to the higher risk of intradialytic hypocalcemia and consequent serious arrhythmias. The calcium levels should be at least 1.5 mmol/L.

The glucose content of the dialysis solution is intended to prevent disequilibrium syndrome by maintaining osmotic pressure in the rapid removal of the urea.

For the preparation of dialysis solutions, purified or ultrapure water is required to relieve almost all impurities. It is prepared in water treatment devices. The initial phase of the adjustment is characterized by filtration (gravel filter of gross impurities, carbon filter, deionizing filter, and others), while the reverse osmosis is used in the second phase. A detailed description of the water treatment processes is not subject and exceeds the scope of my work.

4 Continuous Renal Replacement Therapy (CRRT)

The three key advantages of CRRT are hemodynamic stability, improved fluid and electrolyte balance, and metabolic stability and homeostasis.

The individual methodologies of continuous renal replacement treatment (CRRT = Continual Renal Replacement Therapy) are particularly suitable for hemodynamically compromised patients with AKI (= Acute Kidney Injury) and multiorgan failure (MOF). They allow a slow and gentle removal of the solutes and fluids, with no large transfer of intravascular fluid and minimize electrolyte disbalance, hypotension, and arrhythmias. Hypotension, which occurs during conventional intermittent hemodialysis, may contribute to other ischemic attacks on the kidneys affected by AKI, which distorts the process of healing and recovery of the function. Uremia is controlled in CRRT better than for IHD in catabolic patients with AKI. Ultrafiltration can be achieved either continuously or as necessary to ensure the need to maintain fluid balance in the patient, where parenteral and enteral nutrition and administration of medicinal products are usually required. During CRRT, it is more reliable to maintain the therapeutic level of medicines. It is possible to continuously remove mediators of inflammation, which contributes to better hemodynamic stability.

The studies conducted have not yet demonstrated significant improvement in mortality compared to intermittent hemodialysis, but studies are not randomized on the other side, and patients with hypotension, cardiac dysfunction, sepsis or hemodynamic instability are usually preferential to the treatment of the CRRT. The increase in clinical experience suggests that critically ill patients with renal failure can be better managed through CRRT than IHD. For acutely ill patients, the methodology of the SLED can be a good option or EDD (Extended Daily Dialysis). (LEVY, 2004 s. 306)

The most commonly used techniques currently include:

- **CVVH** (*Continuous venovenous Hemofiltration*) - Continuous veno-venous hemofiltration,

- **CVVHD** (*Continuous venovenous Hemodialysis*) – Continuous veno-venous hemodialysis,

- **CVVHDF** (*Continuous venovenous Hemodiafiltration*) – Continuous veno-venous hemodiafiltration,

- **CAVH** (*Continuous arteriovenous Hemofiltration*) – Continuous arterial-venous hemofiltration,

- **CAVHD** (*Continuous arteriovenous Hemodialysis*) – Continuous arterial-venous hemodialysis,

- **CAVHDF** (*Continuous arteriovenous Hemodiafiltration*) - Continuous arterial-venous hemodiafiltration,

- **SCUF** (*Slow Continuous Ultrafiltration*) – Slow ongoing ultrafiltration,

- **SLED/EDD** (*Sustained Low-Efficiency Dialysis/Extended Daily Dialysis*) - Continuous dialysis with low efficacy/extended daily dialysis.

The care of adult patients' methodologies carried out by the blood pump as part of the monitor for the implementation of CRRT methods predominated over historically older arterio-venous methodologies, where the patient's systemic blood pressure was used as a driving pressure in the extracorporeal circulation. The biggest disadvantage of arterio-venous techniques is the need for arterial access, which is the most common cause of morbidity.

There are no controlled comparisons between hemofilters, and most of the nephrologists and intensivists have experience with only one or two methodologies. Hemofiltration relies on the continuous removal of the solutes and fluids due to the pressure differential to the membrane (effective pressure gradient), while hemodialysis is mainly achieved by the diffusive removal of the solutes. Diffusion is very effective only in removing molecules with a small relative molecular weight, while ultrafiltration eliminates all plasma molecules passing through a high permeable membrane, regardless of their relative molecular weight. Hemodynamic stability is better maintained by the convection transport of the solutes against diffusion for unknown reasons. Hemofiltration does not require dialysis but requires accurate intravenous replacement of the removed fluid volumes, either before or after the filter (predilution or postdilution ways). Controlled Survival Studies in CRRT and IHD are not of large numbers, and most of them showed a significant trend to improve survival during the use of CRRT. Only one study showed the benefit of hemodialysis. (LEVY, 2004 s. 308)

In the sequence/EDD, the conventional hemodialysis device (monitor) and blood flow from 100 to 200 mL/min, the flow of dialysis only 100 mL/min for 8-24 hours are used. Special equipment for the implementation of CRRT methods is required.

The indication of the individual CRRT methods is determined primarily after an assessment of the patient's overall clinical condition. Sometimes the indications are divided into renal (exemplary ones) and extra-renal (potential ones), but the use of indications of CRRT is still questionable. Indication for CRRT also represents the overrun of certain laboratory values. In practice indications are used according to Bellomo and Ronco, namely:

Hyperkaliemia	>	6.5	mmol/L
pH	<	7.1	
Serum Urea	>	30	mmol/L
Serum creatinine	>	500	mmol/L
Serum sodium	<	115	mmol/L or
	>	160	mmol/L

(BELLOMO, 1998)

4.1 Parameters used in CRRT

Clearance of the procedure depends on the type of membrane, blood flow and the size of ultrafiltration. Clearance of urea ranges from 1.7 mL/min at SCUF, over 17 mL/min When CVVH to 30 mL/min for CVVHDF. For comparison in the implementation of IHD three times a week, the weekly clearance of 150 liters, IHD daily about 300 – 350 liter while CRRT is a week 100 liters for PD about 70 liters for a week.

In CRRT methodologies, blood flow from 100 to 150 mL/min is used (somewhere up to 150 – 200 mL/min), dialysis solution flow rate 16 – 33 mL/min or 1 – 2 L/hour well as the flow of dialysis solution and ultrafiltration should be at least 35 mL/kg/h. Anticoagulant is given after patients clinical condition and according to the APTT-R values, which should be extended by 25-50%. To limit the risk of blood clotting in dialyzer (hemofilter, hemodiafilter, eventually hemodialyzer), the ratio of the rate of ultrafiltration and blood flow should be below 20%. In the case of intermittent post-diluent hemofiltration or hemodiafiltration, it is recognized as opposed to CRRT to 30-33%.

4.2 Vascular access for the implementation of CRRT

As vascular access, the CRRT methodologies use the double-lumen intravascular catheter or two single-lumen catheters introduced into the vena jugular interna (internal jugular vein) or to the femoral vein. We strive to avoid access through the subclavian vein because of the risk of subsequent subclavian stenosis. In the internal jugular vein, the position of the catheter is radiologically checked. Standard is the ultrasound-guided insertion. Implanted tunneled catheters may reduce the risk of infection, but in the case of a patient hospitalized in an intensive care unit (ICU) it is more difficult to implement, the procedure is time-consuming and staff-dependent. The need to create an artificial an arterial-venous short-circuit, so-called Scribner's shunt in order to gain access to the implementation of the CRRT method is extremely rare and should be inadequate and inappropriate. Complications are like those of intermittent methods. Catheters should generally be changed every 4-5 days or even before infection or thrombosis occurs.

4.3 Membranes and ultrafiltration achieved in CRRT

CRRT methodologies use high-permeable or high-flux membranes, usually synthetic, which satisfy the requirements of hemofiltration for membrane permeability. The comparison of biocompatibility and incompatibilities in CRRT has resulted in controversial results as regards patient survival and renal function recovery after AKI (LEVY, 2004 s. 310). Over time the membrane is lost as a result of the adsorption of proteins. Therefore it is recommended to exchange hemofilter at least once every 48 hours, better once every 24 hours or according to the current condition.

Ultrafiltration is controlled by volumetric control in view of the need to ensure high accuracy of measurement. The

CAVH is adjusted only by changing the position of the filter bag relative to hemofilter. Volume (volumetric) control relies on the filter pump. In order to achieve adequate removal of the solvent for convection transport, minimum fluid removal at a level of 10- 15 liters per day should be achieved. Depending on the condition of the patient's hydration, most of this fluid is usually replaced by a replacement solution. One controlled study showed worse results in ultrafiltration of 20 mL/kg/h compared to UF 35 to 45 mL/kg/equivalent to 1.35, 2.4 to 2.9 liter per hour). (LEVY, 2004 s. 310)

4.4 Dialysis and replacement solutions for CRRT

The dialysis and substitution (replacement) solution are usually supplied in bags containing 5 liters. Its composition is like that of IHD, but as the buffer system, the lactate is usually used. Citrate is not used yet. When using a separate infusion or in newer systems with separate compartments in a bag, bicarbonate can also be used. In the case of a separate infusion, bicarbonate (8.4% sodium bicarbonate solution) is administered to the central vein in a quantity of 20 to 40 mL per hour. The composition of the solutions is as follows:

Sodium (Natrium)	132 – 140	mmol/L
Potassium (Kalium)	0 – 2	mmol/L
Calcium	1.6 – 1.8	mmol/L
Magnesium (Magnesia)	0.5 – 1.5	mmol/L
Chlorides	100 – 115	mmol/L
Lactate	30 – 45	mmol/L

Lactate-free solutions are hyponatremic (to 110 mmol/L), with the remainder of sodium infused with bicarbonate.

Patients with liver disease (impaired liver function) and pre-existing lactate acidosis should receive lactate-free solutions as they lack the ability to metabolize the lactate for bicarbonate. Bicarbonate solutions provide excellent control of acidosis and should become the preferred choice of.

Conventional solutions for peritoneal dialysis can be used both as dialysis and replacement (substitution) solutions. The glucose present provides approximately 1300 to 2400 kcal per day.

Replacement solutions may be given either before or after the filter (predilution or postdilution), but in high volume CVVH (HV-CVVH), both are administered simultaneously. The risk of post-dilution administration of the substitution solution is the risks of the rise of hematocrit inside the capillary of hemofilter and the consequent blood clotting in hemofilter, which should avoid adherence to the ratio of total ultrafiltration to the blood flow to 20%. The predilution reduces the concentration of waste solutes in hemofilter but does not significantly reduce their clearance (only partially, marginally). The design of the latest hemofilters allows the so-called middle dilution (mid-dilution). During the execution of

CRRT, there is also a considerable loss of amino acids at level 1 to 5 g per day.

4.5 Anticoagulation during CRRT

Blood clotting in extracorporeal circulation is a major problem, but continuous anticoagulation increases significantly the risk of bleeding (occurs in up to 25% of patients). Predisposed factors of thrombosis in extracorporeal circulation in CRRT are:

1. Use of arterio-venous technique (due to reliance on blood pressure of the patient).

2. Use of capillary dialyzer (and not parallel plate dialyzer). But plate dialyzers are almost not used at present.

3. Problems with the dialysis catheter.

4. Increased ultrafiltration values (UF).

5. Low blood flow values (Q_B).

6. Post-dilutive delivery of the replacement solution (postdilution).

7. Reduced levels of antithrombin-III in critically ill patients with acute renal failure.

Hemofilter should withstand 24 – 36 hours. Polyacrylonitrile filters have a higher frequency of blood clotting in hemofilter than polyamide filters. It is worth to start carrying out the CRRT methodology without using heparin and use it only if blood clotting occurs in hemofilter in less than 24 hours.

To monitor blood clotting in extracorporeal circulation, perform:

> ➢ Visual control of the extracorporeal circuit including the arterial and venous balloon for the presence of blood clots;

> ➢ Regular measurement of APTT-R and Quick Time in INR when using unfractionated heparin;

> ➢ Regular control of anti-Xa levels when using fractionated low-molecular heparin (LMWH) and danaparoid;

> ➢ Regular control of the Quick Time in INR and calcium levels when using sodium citrate to prevent clotting.

4.5.1 *Heparin (unfractionated heparin)*

Heparin is the most commonly used anticoagulant substance. It adds within of the flushing solution in the quantity of 1000 to 3000 units (IU = International Unit) per liter of saline. Sometimes it may be possible to meet the indication of the quantity of heparin in grams. One gram of heparin corresponds then to 100 IU of heparin (1g = 100 IU). By default, the initial bolus dose of 2000 to 5000 units is used and the subsequent continuous infusion of heparin with a speed of 300 to 800 units per hour to the arterial set. The dilution of heparin allows its better mixing with blood. The risk of bleeding can be limited by monitoring the value of APTT-R and the Quick's time in INR (International Normalized Ratio). Blood clotting occurs more often as a result of "mechanical" problems than due to low anticoagulation.

The regional administration of heparin is performed by administration prior to the filter and neutralization of heparin by the protamine sulfate after the filter. 1 mg of protamine sulfate neutralizes the effect of approximately 100 units of heparin (1 g of unfractionated heparin and approx. 60% of this amount in LMWH). The need for rigorous monitoring is inevitable. This method is not used frequently also due to possible serious adverse reactions of protamine sulfate such as anaphylactoid reactions, hypotension, leukopenia, and thrombocytopenia. Protamine sulfate remains in reserve to block the effects of heparin in severe systemic bleeding.

4.5.2 Low-molecular heparins (LMWH), fractionated

Low-molecular heparin may provide less risk of bleeding and a better prediction of the anticoagulant effect, as well as a lower incidence of thrombocytopenia. Usually, it is used 2000 to 3000 units of anti-Xa LMWH every 20 minutes or 35 IU/kg as the initial bolus, and then continuous 13 IU/kg for an hour in the infusion. It can be monitored by measuring the anti-factor X activity. The target values are:

➢ 0.5 - 1 IU/mL in patients without bleeding risk;

➢ 0.2 – 0.4 IU/mL in patients at risk of bleeding.

The use of low-molecular heparin can be combined with prostacyclin (PGI_2) in patients with thrombocytopenia-induced heparin, or fondaparinux use is possible.

4.5.3 Implementation of CRRT without anticoagulation

The use of anticoagulant is not recommended in patients with blood clotting disorders, thrombocytopenia, recent bleeding and liver diseases. In careful management, the hemofilter should withstand more than 24 hours. Hemodiafiltration with predilution and higher blood flow carries a lesser risk of blood clotting in the extracorporeal circuit and hemofilter. Intermittent flushing of the extracorporeal radius of approx. 200 – 300 milliliters of physiological solution can significantly help. If heparin is not completely contraindicated, it can be used at least in the solution for flushing of the circuit prior to initiating the procedure, or a higher dosage of heparin should be used in the saline solution for rinsing up to a value of 20 000 units of heparin.

4.5.4 Regional anticoagulants with sodium citrate

The regional use of sodium citrate ensure that no systemic signs of anticoagulants are manifested, it maintains the excellent lifetime of the filters, there is minimal risk of bleeding, but it requires careful monitoring, separate calcium infusion, and non-standard replacement solutions.

Citrate binds calcium from the blood, thus inhibiting several steps of the hemocoagulation cascade. When returned to the patient, its effect is neutralized by binding large amounts of calcium in the patient's bloodstream, and the liver metabolizes it to bicarbonate. In order to avoid hypocalcemia, a continuous calcium infusion must be administered. Replacement (substitution) and dialysis solutions must not contain calcium. If all these conditions are met, this is a whole successful method.

Example regimen setting:

- ➤ 4% sodium citrate is infused into the arterial access of the hemofiltration circuit (dilution: 90 mL of 46.7% sodium citrate to 1000 mL of 5% glucose solution);

- ➤ 0.75% Calcium chloride solution is infused to the patient's central venous access (dilution: 80 mL of 10% calcium chloride to 1000 mL of a normal physiological solution - saline);

- ➤ The sodium citrate solution is administered at a rate of 190 mL per hour and a replacement calcium solution at a rate of 60 mL per hour;

- ➤ The calcium level in the circuit and the level of ionized calcium in the systemic bloodstream of the patient is monitored at least every hour until these levels are not stable, and then every 4 to 6 hours, maintained at a value of 0.25-0.35 mmol/L in the extracorporeal (extra-body) circuit and 0.9-1.2 mmol/L of ionized calcium in the system circulation;

- ➤ The infusion of the citrate is titrated according to the calcium levels in the extracorporeal (extra-body) circuit;

> The calcium infusion is titrated according to systemic ionized calcium levels.

In addition, patients should be monitored for potential alkalosis, hypocalcemia, and hypernatremia. Infusion of citrate and calcium solutions must be stopped if blood flow or dialysis solution flow are stopped for more than 10 minutes.

This method of anticoagulation should not be used if the patient has liver disease or because of severe alkalosis. (LEVY, 2004 s. 320)

4.5.5 Other options for anticoagulation in CRRT

Prostacyclin (PGI_2) inhibits platelet aggregation and adhesion and acts as a vasodilator. The antiplatelet activity lasts for 2 hours. It is used at a dose of 4 – 8 ng/kg/min. Studies showed a low efficacy when it was administered separately but in combination with low-dosing heparin or LMWH, extended lifetime of filters has been demonstrated. Prostacyclin may cause blood pressure decreases predominantly due to its vasodilatation effect.

Danaparoid (Orgaran) is low molecular weight glucosamine and can be used in patients with thrombocytopenia-induced by heparin (HIT). When used, there is a high risk of bleeding, and despite everything, it may also induce thrombocytopenia. It is used as a bolus in the introduction of 2500 IU with a subsequent infusion 400-600 IU/h for the first 4 hours, while the dose is then reduced to 200-600 IU/h in order to maintain the anti-Xa levels 0.5-1 IU/mL

Other options are to use nafamostat mesylate (a serine protease inhibitor) and recombinant hirudin, which can be seen in all CRRT methodologies, but rarely used.

4.6 Possible complications in CRRT

The CRRT methodologies are generally well tolerated with a similar incidence of complications than the standard IHD, but a lower incidence is recorded.

A great part of them consists of the complications associated with vascular access. These are mainly thrombosis (in the catheter or in the vein), injection site hemorrhage, infections (injection sites, bacteremia, sepsis – especially Gram-positive microorganisms), recirculation (for veno-venous techniques) and insufficient blood flow (wrapping, thrombosis).

There may also be precipitation, blood loss (accidental separation of the circuit, blood clotting in the circuit), sepsis, circuit disconnection, excessive ultrafiltration, fluid, and allergic/hypersensitivity reactions (for plastics, hemofilter or sterilization agents).

In the use of anticoagulant, local or systemic bleeding may occur, thrombocytopenia (especially the development of a HIT in the use of heparin), alkalosis or hypokalemia (regional anticoagulant citrate).

Other possible complications are hypothermia, hypotension, arrhythmia, electrolyte imbalance (hypophosphatemia, hypokalemia, hypocalcemia, hypo or hypernatremia), alkalosis, bio-incompatibilities, air embolism, interactions with ACE inhibitors, loss of nutrients (amino acids and trace elements). The dosage of medicines is different from the intermittent hemodialysis too.

5 Hepatic Dialysis – Detoxifying Artificial Hepatic Supportive Therapy

Mortality in acute liver failure (ALF) remains high despite intensive supportive care. Mortality values range from 60% to 90% depending on the cause of the liver disease itself. In Western Europe, the survival of patients with ALF caused by acute hepatitis B is 12% to 23% (BERNUAU, 1986). From the fifties of the 20th century, some methodologies were used to help the failing liver. This was a range of different treatments from the treatment with medicaments and pills to the therapy of Liver Support Equipment ("Liver Support Devices") and liver transplantation. Currently, the standard treatment with ALF is the orthotopic liver transplantation (OLT = Orthotopic Liver Transplantation). Urgent OLT is associated with one year's survival in 60% to 90% of patients depending on the cause of ALF and the selection criteria used for OLT (FARMER, 2003).

However, due to the lack of liver organ donors, a significant number of patients with ALF die during the period of inclusion in the waiting list on the OLT. Despite efforts to increase the numbers of liver donations from donors for example by using divided seals, living relatives of the liver and using the marginal organs, there are much fewer liver organs available than the need for OLT.

Due to the high levels of mortality and prolonged waiting times for transplantation in recent years (United Network for Organ Sharing, 2009), again the interest in techniques that allow temporary support of the liver function to overcome the period when the patient with ALF waits for OLT or to regenerate the liver revives. In general, these techniques can be divided into two primary groups.

5.1 Non-biological liver support

Low and medium relative molecular weight toxic substances play a decisive role in ALF. These in water soluble and protein-bound toxins cause multiorgan failure and hepatic encephalopathy, leading to coma and possible death. Many attempts have been undertaken ensuring the patient's blood detoxification will be appropriate to develop non-biological liver support.

The system of extracorporeal support for the liver should/must provide a positive and major liver function:

1. Detoxification.
2. Synthesis.
3. Regulation.

Understanding the fact that the critical point of the clinical picture in liver failure is the accumulating toxins, which are not removed by the failing liver, led to the development of artificial filtration and adsorption devices. Based on this hypothesis, the removal of lipophilic agents bound to the albumin such as bilirubin, bile acids, aromatic amino acid metabolites, fatty acids with the middle-chain, cytokines, and others may help to the clinical progress in a patient with liver failure. (https://en.wikipedia.org/wiki/Liver_dialysis)

Renal failure is usually replaced by hemodialysis, but it has limited use in liver failure because it does not remove albumin-bound toxins. Artificial detoxification devices, which are currently clinically evaluated, include 1. Molecular adsorption recirculating system [Molecular Adsorbent Recirculating System (MARS)], 2. Dialysis with a single pass of albumin [Single-Pass Albumin Dialysis (SPAD)] and 3. Prometheus System®.

In the fifties of the last century, the use of the hemodialysis to remove toxins began, but no improvement was achieved in the survival. Hemofiltration, i.e., continuous cautious removal of the solutes by shifting them through a semi-permeable membrane, also achieved limited results. Improvement in survival has not been achieved using hemoperfusion and plasma perfusion, thus more aggressive by eliminating protein-bound toxic molecules. Different types of elimination were used, which were particularly effective in the removal of lipid a protein bound substance. Significant experience has been gained when using activated coal as an adsorbent of possible toxins. Finally, however, the conclusions of the studies audited showed that these techniques did not improve survival. Hemadsorption, dialysis in combination with activated carbon and cation inverter, improved biochemical parameters, the clinical condition of the patient, but it did not improved survival. Non-specific targeting of the technology was considered the cause of this limited success. In summary, in this period the hemodialysis, hemofiltration, high-volume plasmapheresis, hemodiafiltration, hemoperfusion, and hemodiabsorption were used.

The most promising non-biological supportive therapies combine detoxification water-soluble and protein-bound toxins in the dialysis system. These are, e.g., the following devices, but other systems are also being developed.

1. MARS – Molecular Adsorption Recirculating System.

2. SPAD = Single Pass Albumin Dialysis.

3. Artificial Liver Support System (ALSS).

4. PF-Liver Dialysis.

5. Prometheus System®.

Several non-biological liver support systems demonstrated their usefulness in the short-term support of the liver in moderately impaired patients with ALF. However, their non-specificity in removing various compounds and their lack of capacity to synthesize proteins specific to the liver and other hepatotropic factors are likely to contribute to their limited efficacy. The success of OLT has again pointed to the importance of not only detoxification but also metabolic functions on positive outcomes for the patient. Since these functions can carry hepatocytes, more is expected from biological liver support systems. (VAN DE KERKHOVE, 2004)

MARS – Molecular adsorption recirculating system [Molecular Adsorbent Recirculating System]

The development of the MARS system began at the University of Rostock in Germany, and it was developed by Teraklin AG in Germany. It is the most famous extracorporeal hepatic dialysis system, and it is here now over 20 years. It consists of two separate dialysis circuits. The first circuit contains the human albumin, which comes into contact with the patient's blood through a semipermeable membrane. It has two special filters to purify the albumin after it absorbed the toxins from the patient's blood. The second circuit consisted of a hemodialysis device and used to clean the albumin in the first circuit before recirculating again to the semipermeable membrane, where it again encounters the patient's blood. MARS can remove many toxins, including ammonia, bile acids, bilirubin, copper, iron, aromatic amino acids, short-and medium-chain fatty acids, tryptophan, creatinine, urea, diazepam, benzodiazepine-like substances, nitrous oxide, phenytoin, and phenols.

SPAD - Dialysis with a Single Pass of Albumin

Dialysis with a one-time switching of albumin is a technically simple method of albumin dialysis, which uses standard treatment devices to replace renal function without the additional perfusion pump system. The patient's blood flows through a range of capillary hemodiafilter with high flow ("high-flux" hemodiafilter), which is identical to that used in the MARS System. The other side of the membrane is filled with the solution in the opposite direction that leaves the filter (goes as biologically hazardous waste). Hemodialysis can be performed in the first circuit through the same "high-flux" capillary
hemodiafilter. (https://en.wikipedia.org/wiki/Liver_dialysis)

Prometheus System®

This is a new device of Fresenius Medical Care based on the combination of albumin adsorption (FPSA Circuit) with high-flux hemodialysis after selective filtration of the albumin fraction through a specific polysulfide filter (Albuflow) (RIFAI, 2003). Its efficacy has been studied in patients with hepatorenal syndrome. Treatment lasting two consecutive days significantly reduced serum levels of conjugated bilirubin, bile acids, ammonia, cholinesterase, creatinine, urea, and improved pH.

5.2 Biological Liver Support

Biological accesses rely on Featured Liver or hepatocytes of xenogeneic or human origin, which is noted to be used to support the patient's liver. These features include detoxification, several metabolic functions, and protein synthesis and other molecules.

In 1956, it was shown that fresh homogenate of the bovine liver could be used for the metabolism of salicylic acid, barbituric acid, and ketone particles and for the formation of urea of ammonium chloride. Many of the different biological practices that followed contained Xeno and cross-hemodialysis in which the patient's blood was dialyzed by the blood of the living animal or animal preparations. However, these technical benefits for patients with hepatic failure were not considered suitable for clinical application due to their complexity of the procedure itself or rapid loss of efficacy. In addition, xenogeneic extracorporeal human liver transplantation has temporarily demonstrated improvements in biochemical parameters and clinical neurologic status of the patient. However, controlled clinical studies showing an improvement in survival are still not available. Liver support can be achieved in humans. Another possibility is the exchange transfusion, which was associated with the reverse of the hepatic coma. In combination with hemodialysis, the survival increased from 18% to 50% (4 of 8 patients) in one uncontrolled study (BRUNNER, 1987). The main problem of exchange transfusions is the need for a large amount of normal plasma.

Isolated liver cells were used in different configurations: suspended, attached to the substrate and encapsulated in semipermeable membranes. Hepatocytes used to support the liver can be divided into two categories, namely implantable systems and extracorporeal systems. A few cases have been reported concerning human transplant hepatocytes with benefit to the patient, but no transplantation of Xenogeneic hepatocytes has been reported yet.

Problems with blood clotting and immune response in extracorporeal perfusion of the liver have led to the development of hybrid liver support devices. BAL systems are extracorporeal systems temporarily attached to the patient's circulation. Bioartificial Liver Systems consists of the artificial component, i.e., Bioreactor and its equipment and from biocomponents, i.e., hepatocytes. At present there is a significant increase and development of various bioartificial hepatic systems, in practice, 11 different BALS installations have been used. (VAN DE KERKHOVE, 2004) Such clinically applied SSA systems include, for example, the following devices:

1. Extracorporeal Liver Assist Device (**ELAD**) – Extra-body (extracorporeal) liver assistance equipment.

2. **Hepatassist** BAL Device -Bioartificial Liver Equipment.

3. Teca-Hybrid Artificial Liver Support System (**Teca-HALSS**) – Hybrid artificial hepatic support system Teca.

4. Bioartificial Liver Support System (**BLSS**).

5. Radial Flow Bioreactor (**RFB**).

6. Hybrid Liver Support System (**HLSS**) and Modular Extracorporeal Liver Support (**MELS**).

7. AMC – Bioartificial Liver (**AMC-BAL**).

8. Bioartificial Hepatic Support System (**BHSS**).

9. Hybrid — Bioartificial Liver (**HBAL**).

The concept of supporting liver function through BAL systems succeed in animal studies. In addition, it has been demonstrated that the clinical use of BALS devices is safe. (CO2 Science) Clinical evaluation of the treatment of individual BALS systems is significantly impeded by significant differences between patient groups as well as the fact that most patients undergo a subsequent OLT. However, neurological and biochemical parameters have improved after treatment with different BALS devices. Research in the field of BAL equipment should concentrate on the exchange of hepatocytes of animal origin for hepatocytes of human origin, whether primary hepatocytes or immortal cell lines, to overcome possible problems and zoonoses. (VAN DE KERKHOVE, 2004)

6 OTHER METHODS OF EXTRACORPOREAL (EXTRA-BODY) ELIMINATION TREATMENT

Other important methods of extracorporeal (extra-body) elimination treatment also apply. **Plasmapheresis** that can be carried out either by the power of ultracentrifugation or in the form of membrane separation of plasma (MPS). For MPS, the separate plasma may be further modified to remove certain types of substances, for example, **Immunoadsorption**, and this can be returned to the patient. In this way, plasmapheresis is largely applied to the treatment of various autoimmune diseases. Diseases that can be used by plasmapheresis include, for example:

1. Guillain-Barré syndrome (Acute inflammatory demyelinating polyneuropathy).

2. Chronic inflammatory demyelinating polyneuropathy (Chronic relapsing polyneuropathy).

3. Goodpasture syndrome.

4. Hyperviscosity syndromes:

    a. Cryoglobulinemia.

b. Paraproteinemia.

   c. Waldenström's macroglobulinemia

5. Myasthenia gravis.

6. Thrombotic thrombocytopenic purpura (TTP)/hemolytic-uremic syndrome (hemolytic anemia, acute renal failure – uremia and thrombocytopenia).

7. Granulomatosis with polyangiitis – Antibodies against acetylcholine receptor on the post-synaptic side of the neuromuscular junction.

8. Lambert-Eaton Syndrome (Autoimmune damage to the calcium channel of the neuromuscular connection).

9. Antiphospholipid syndrome (APL) – Autoimmune hemocoagulation disorder, antibodies to phospholipids (APL) as a component of cell membranes characterized by the presence of anti-cardiolipin antibodies and β2-glycoprotein I and causes abortion, premature birth of the fetus or severe preeclampsia.

10. Microscopic polyangiitis.

11. Recurrent focal and segmental glomerulosclerosis in the transplanted kidney.

12. HELLP syndrome (Variant preeclampsia – hemolytic anemia, elevated hepatic enzymes, thrombocytopenia).

13. Refsum's disease (Heredopathia Atactica Polyneuritiformis) – Malformations of myelin, peroxisome disease.

14. Bechet's syndrome – A form of vasculitis leading to ulcerations and lesions.

15. Neuropathies associated with HIV infection (KIPROV, 1992).

16. Graves' disease in children and neonates.

17. Pemphigus Vulgaris.

Immunoadsorption can eliminate large amounts of immunoglobulins from Patient circulation with minimal side effects known from plasma. Unlike it, the mere conventional plasma exchange removes antibodies and other plasma factors in the range of 50-75% (KELLER, 1983). Immunoglobulins are distributed in intravascular and extravascular space in approximately the same amount. The inflammatory process often takes place in tissue and not in the vascular bed. The easy removal of immunoglobulins from circulation may, in any case, affect the cessation of the immune process. Repeated cycles with adequately processed plasma volumes must be used to overcome the redistribution of pathological autoantibodies. It seems that concomitant administration of intravenous immunoglobulins weakens the effect of adsorption of immunoglobulins in certain circumstances than for lupus erythematosus, although both two treatments have been shown to be both effective itself. (BRAUN, 1999). The point is that extensive immunoadsorption to achieve the desired effect on the humoral immune system, which would exceed the effect of separate plasmapheresis (BRAUN, 1998). Despite almost complete IgG elimination, it results in severe humoral immune deficiency and, in clinical practice, attention must be given to any infectious complication.

Immunoadsorption devices can be divided into non-selective, semi-selective and highly selective adsorbers. Non-selective adsorbers (dextrose-sulfate, tryptophan, and phenylalanine) reduce the plasma levels of many different substances such as fibrinogen, albumin, lipids, and immunoglobulins. Semiselective adsorbers (staphylococcal protein A, anti-human Ig adsorber) exhibit an affinity for only one group of plasma proteins. Highly selective adsorbers eliminate specific substances without altering the blood levels of other plasma components. Technically, single-use adsorbers or absorbers are available for re-use. (BRAUN, 1998)

Another of the different methods of extracorporeal (extra-body) elimination treatment is an LDL-apheresis, a form of apheresis imitating dialysis technique designed to eliminate particles of low-density lipoproteins containing cholesterol (LDL-cholesterol). Used in rare homozygote familial hypercholesterolemia if it is not possible to correct by the normal medicaments' treatment and similar diseases. Length of the procedure is 2 – 4 hours, and it is repeated several times a week to keep LDL levels at a low level and avoid cardiovascular disease. This is a financially demanding procedure limited to certain severe cases of hyperlipidemia.

The principle of LDL-apheresis is the passage of blood through the column covered by antibodies against apolipoprotein B, dextrose-sulphate or polyacrylate, possibly by precipitating LDL heparin at low pH. In all cases (except polyacrylate absorption), the plasma is first separated from the cells by the method of membrane separation of plasma. An example is the use of the Liposorber® device from Kaneka.

In the future, further developments and discoveries of other new methods can be achieved in the extracorporeal (extra-body) elimination treatment, which will both detect new areas of their medical application. It is reasonable to expect the application and further improvement of already known methods and medical benefits from the development.

The question, on the other hand, remains the financial coverage of these costly treatment methods.

LIST OF USED LITERATURE

BELLOMO, R. - RONCO, C. 1998. Indications and criteria for initiating renal replacement therapy in the intensive care unit. 1998, Vol. Suppl.66, 53, pp. 106-109.

BERNUAU, J. - RUEFF, B. - BENHAMOU, J.P. 1986. Fulminant and subfulminant liver failure: definitions and causes. 1986, 6, pp. 97-106.

BORG, Frank. 2003. *What is osmosis? Explanation and understanding of a physical phenomenon.* Karleby : Jyväskylä University, Chydenius Institute, 2003. Accessible at http://arxiv.org/abs/physics/0305011v1.

BRAUN, N. - KADAR, J.G. - RISLER, T. 1998. Therapeutic immunoadsorption - its role in clinical practice. *Transfus.Sci.* 1998, 19, pp. 65-69.

BRAUN, N. - RISLER, T. 1999. Immunoadsorption as a tool for the immunomodulation of the humoral and cellular immune system in autoimmune disease. *Ther.Apher.* 1999, 3, pp. 240-245.

BRUNNER, G. - LOSGEN, H. 1987. Benefits and dangers of plasma with fulminant hepatic failure. [book auth.] T. - SHIOKAWA, Y. - INOUE, N. ODA. *Therapeutic plasmapheresis VI.* Cleveland, Ohio : ISAO Press, 1987, pp. 187-191.

CONSTANZO, M. R. - SALTZBERG, M. T. 2007. *Ultrafiltration versus intravenous diuretics for patients hospitalized for acutely decompensated heart failure.* 2007. pp. 675-83. Vol. 6, Accessible at http://www.ncbi.nlm.nih.gov/pubmed/17291932 Citované dňa 29.marca 2009..

DE FRANCISCO, ALM. - PINERA, C. - HERAS, M. et al. 2000. Hemodiafiltration with On-Line Endogenous Reinfusion. 2000, 18, pp. 231-236.

EISELT, J. 2002. Hemofiltrace a hemomdiafiltrace. 2002, 8, pp. 103-109.

FARMER, D.G. - ANSELMO, D.M. - GHOBRIAL, R.M. et al. 2003. Liver transplantation for fulminant hepatic failure: experience with more than 200 patients over a 17-year period. 2003, 237, pp. 666-676.

HARDY, James K. 2003. Botany online: Membranes and Transport - Osmosis. *www.biologie.uni-hamburg.de*. [Online] Peter v. Sengbusch, 7 31, 2003. [Cited: 3 27, 2009.] http://www.biologie.uni-hamburg.de/b-online/e22/22c.htm.

HAYNIE, Donald T. 2001. *Biological Thermodynamics.* Cambridge : Cambridge University Press, 2001.

KADLEC, Oskár a kol. 1997. *Encyklopédia medicíny.* [ed.] CSc MUDr. Oskár Kadlec. Bratislava : Asclepios, 1997. pp. 181-183. Vol. V. 80-7167-013-8.

KELLER, F. - WAGNER, K. - FABER, U. - SCHOLLE, J. - NEUMAYER, H. H. - MAIGA, M. - SCHULTZE, G. - OFFERMANN, G. - MOLZAHN, M. 1983. Elimination kinetics of plasma exchange. *Klin. Wochenschr.* 1983, 61, pp. 1115-1122.

KIPROV, D.D. - STRICKER, R.B. - MILLER, R.G. 1992. Treatment of HIV neuropathy with plasmapheresis and intravenous gammaglobulin. *Int Conf AIDS.* Jul 19-24, 1992, 8.

LEVY, Jeremy - MORGAN, Julie - BROWN, Edwina. 2004. *Oxford handbook of dialysis.* Second edition. Oxford : Oxford University Press, 2004. 0-19-852954-6.

LOPOT, František. 2000. Hemodialyzační technika. [book auth.] Sylvie SULKOVÁ. *Hemodialýza*. Praha : MAXDORF - JESSENIUS®, 2000.

MATON, Anthea - HOPKINS, Jean - JOHNSON, Susan - LAHART, David - WARNER, Maryanna Quon - WRIGHT, Jill D. 1997. *Cells Building Blocks of Life*. New Jersey : Prentice Hall, 1997.

MYDLÍK, Miroslav. 2004. Eliminačné metódy v liečbe chronickej renálnej insuficiencie. [book auth.] Rastislav - ŠAŠINKA, Miroslav - MYDLÍK, Miroslav - KOVÁCS, László DZÚRIK. *Nefrológia*. Dieškova edícia. Bratislava : Herba, 2004, Vol. 1, pp. 752-757.

OPATRNÝ, Karel - POLAKOVIČ, Vladimír. 2006. Mimotělní metody nahrazující funkci ledvin. [book auth.] Vladimír a kol. TEPLAN. *Praktická nefrologie*. Praha : Grada Publishing, a.s., 2006, 16, pp. 385-406.

PANICHI, V. - DE PIETRO, S. - ANDREINI, B. et al. 1998. Cytokine production in haemodiafiltration: a multicentre study. 1998, 13, pp. 1737-1744.

PHILIBERT, Jean. 2005. *Diffusion-Fundamentals. The Open-Access Journal for the Basic Principles of Diffusion Theory, Experiment, and Application*. [Online] 2005. [Dátum: 27. Marec 2009.] http://www.uni-leipzig.de/diffusion/journal/pdf/volume2/diff_fund-2(2005)1.pdf.

RIFAI, K. - ERNST, T. - KRETSCHMER, U. - BAHR, M.J. - SCHNEIDER, A. - HAFER, C. - HALLER, H. - MANNS, M.P. - FLISER, D. 2003. Prometheus - a new extracorporeal system for the treatment of liver failure. *J Hepatol*. December 2003, Vol. 6, 39, pp. 984-990.

STEDDON, Simon - ASHMAN, Neil - CHESSER, Alistair - CUNNINGHAM, John. 2006. *Oxford Handbook of Nephrology and Hypertension*. Oxford

Handbooks. New York : Oxford University Press Inc, 2006. ISBN 0-19-852069-7.

SULKOVÁ, Sylvie. 2000. Základní principy hemodialýzy. [book auth.] Sylvie a kol. SULKOVÁ. *Hemodialýza*. Praha : MAXDORF - JESSENIUS®, 2000, 4.

TESAŘ, Vladimír - SCHÜCK, Otto a kol. 2006. *Klinická nefrologie*. Praha : Grada Publishing, a.s., 2006. 80-247-0503-6.

United Network for Organ Sharing. 2009. Liver transplantation data 2002. *www.unos.org*. [Online] United Network for Organ Sharing, 2009. [Cited: 4 4, 2009.] http://www.unos.org/.

URSELL, Tristan S. 2007. The Diffusion Equation. A Multi-dimensional Tutorial. *www.rpgroup.caltech.edu*. [Online] Department of Applied Physics, California Institute of Technology, October 2007. [Cited: 3 27, 2009.] http://www.rpgroup.caltech.edu/~natsirt/aph162/diffusion.pdf.

VAN DE KERKHOVE, Maarten Paul - HOEKSTRA, Ruurdtje - CHAMULEAU, Robert A. F. M. - VAN GULIK, Thomas M. 2004. Clinical Application of Bioartificial Liver Support Systems. *Annals of Surgery*. August 2004, Vol. 240, 2, pp. 216-230.

Wikipedia. The Free Encyclopedia. Adsorption. 2009. Adsorption. *en.wikipedia.org*. [Online] Wikipedia. The Free Encyclopedia, 3 22, 2009. [Cited: 3 29, 2009.] http://en.wikipedia.org/wiki/Adsorption.

Wikipedia. The Free Encyclopedia. Colligative properties. 2009. Colligative properties. *en.wikipedia.org*. [Online] Wikipedia. The Free Encyclopedia., 3 21, 2009. [Cited: 3 27, 2009.] http://en.wikipedia.org/wiki/Colligative_properties.

Wikipedia. The Free Encyclopedia. Fick's law of diffusion. 2009. Fick's law of diffusion. *en.wikipedia.org.* [Online] Wikipedia. The Free Encyclopedia, 3 11, 2009. [Cited: 3 27, 2009.] http://en.wikipedia.org/wiki/Fick%27s_law_of_diffusion.

Wikipedia. The Free Encyclopedia. Molecular diffusion. 2009. Molecular diffusion. *en.wikipedia.org.* [Online] Wikipedia. The Free Encyclopedia., 3 12, 2009. [Cited: 3 27, 2009.] http://en.wikipedia.org/wiki/Molecular_diffusion.

Wikipedia. The Free Encyclopedia. Osmosis. 2009. Osmosis. *en.wikipedia.org.* [Online] Wikipedia. The Free Encyclopedia., 3 26, 2009. [Cited: 3 27, 2009.] http://en.wikipedia.org/wiki/Osmosis.

Wikipedia. The Free Encyclopedia. Reverse osmosis. 2009. Reverse osmosis. *en.wikipedia.org.* [Online] Wikipedia. The Free Encyclopedia., 3 19, 2009. [Cited: 3 27, 2009.] http://en.wikipedia.org/wiki/Reverse_osmosis.

Lubomir Polascin: Blood Purification. 2019.

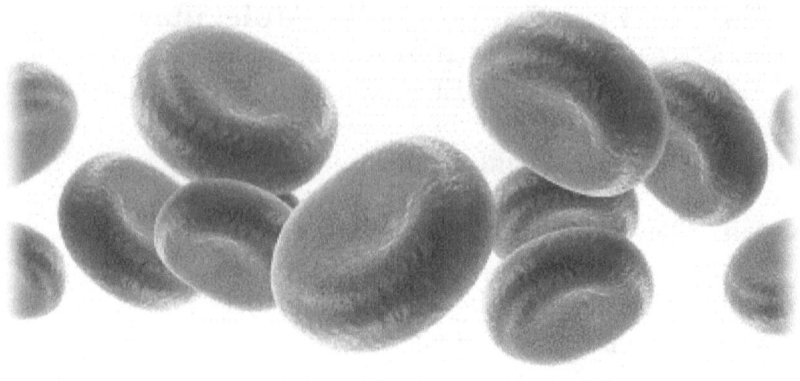

The End

www.ingramcontent.com/pod-product-compliance
Lightning Source LLC
Chambersburg PA
CBHW021820170526
45157CB00007B/2657